FATHERING
Participation in labor and birth

FATHERING

Participation in labor and birth

CELESTE R. PHILLIPS, R.N., M.S.

Instructor, Mission College,
West Valley Joint Community College District,
Saratoga, California

JOSEPH T. ANZALONE, M.D.

Director, Joseph T. Anzalone Foundation,
Santa Cruz, California

with 73 illustrations

The C. V. Mosby Company

Saint Louis   1978

The C.V. Mosby Company
11830 Westline Industrial Drive, St. Louis, Missouri 63141

Library of Congress Cataloging in Publication Data

Phillips, Celeste R   1933-
    Fathering: participation in labor and birth.

    Bibliography: p.
    1. Pregnancy. 2. Childbirth. 3. Fathers.
I. Anzalone, Joseph T., 1931-   joint author.
II. Title.
RG525.P448   618.4   77-13224
ISBN 0-8016-3919-0

TS/M/M 9 8 7 6 5 4 3 2 1

TO
OUR FATHERS

Preface

To many people in our culture, parenthood means motherhood. This book focuses primarily on the father of the family and his involvement with labor and birth—an aspect of parenthood that has received too little attention in the past. We do not intend to underestimate the mother's role or to attack motherhood. We are simply saying that fathers are important, too, and are making a plea for recognition of the father as a vital, interacting member of the family.

This book is written as a supplemental text for maternity nursing courses, obstetrical courses in medical schools, family-life classes, and parenting classes. Childbirth educators will also use this book to share information regarding fathers with parents and future parents.

Nursing and medical literature relating to fathers' involvement during pregnancy and birth has been sparse, and countless textbooks do not even have "father" listed in their index.

On reviewing the psychological literature, it appears that the American male's parental role is almost limited to impregnation, paying bills nine months later, and then magically appearing again as a role model for adolescent boys. Furthermore, much of the work of sociologists and anthropologists, who have contributed most to the literature on fathers, is only observational.

On the other hand, much information can be found in texts relative to the importance of the father's understanding all physiological and psychological changes of the woman during pregnancy. Although again and again he is encouraged to help her, support her, anticipate her needs, and understand her, little is written regarding his needs.

Newspaper articles on pregnancy, childbirth, and parenthood are usually relegated to the women's page, and information articles on all aspects of parenting are traditionally found only in women's magazines. Books on pregnancy and birth for parents are almost always addressed to the mother, with occasional references to the father in a supportive role of some kind.

Researchers frequently explain that their studies are mother centered because the father was not available for interview as a result of his work schedule or obligations outside the home. This lack of information on fathers and fathering has further reinforced the idea that fathers in our culture are not interested in birth or in babies.

After all, we can see the mother's physiological changes: enlarged abdomen, swelling breasts, changing posture, and obvious protective mechanisms as she adapts to the growing fetus within her. Furthermore, we can even see the way she gives birth, suckles the child at her breasts, and actively cares for the child's needs. Granted, a mother for the first time has to learn her role, but her physiology helps her reinforce reality and even trigger her feelings. The role of the father is also learned, but there are no visible, significant physical changes in the father in pregnancy.

The traditional father role accepted by our culture is that of the manly breadwinner. Should a man express tender, nurturing feelings and be interested and totally involved in pregnancy and birth, he may be considered an invader in a woman's world. Since fathers tend to be undervalued in our culture, we propose that men may have suffered as much from discrimination as have women—particularly when it comes to pregnancy and birth. Times are changing, however, and many men are seriously pondering on their roles as fathers and are expressing dissatisfaction with the one assigned to them by our culture. These same men are attempting to reject exaggerated definitions of masculinity and femininity and to redefine their sex roles from rigid, stereotyped terms to more human terms. As part of this changing philosophy, many of these men, as they become fathers, involve themselves by participating actively throughout pregnancy and birth, and although the numbers are still small, their philosophy is spreading.

One look at our dramatically reduced maternal and infant mortality and morbidity in the past fifty years emphasizes that the practice of medicine in the United States has come a long way and is worthy of pride. However, medical education and training are often more scientific than human, and in our effort to reduce the infection rate in maternity units, what has happened to the father?

The role of the father in a modern hospital maternity setting is often uncertain. Often he is allowed to remain only on the fringes of the childbearing experience, tolerated as a necessary nuisance, relegated to the "Fathers' Waiting Room," and assigned to a particular chair or place out of the way. In many hospitals the father is excluded from the labor room when the woman is medicated and then excluded from the delivery room as well. Is it any wonder that we still know little of men's experiences and feelings during pregnancy and birth?

Although many hospitals still treat fathers as excess baggage, increasingly more hospitals are promoting father participation, inviting him to childbirth preparation classes and accepting him at the birth. With this book we are making a plea for support of these institutions which are changing and for a rethinking by the medical profession and the public of the father's role in pregnancy and birth. We believe that the couple should be enriched both physically and emotionally by the childbirth experience, not only surviving childbirth well but also becoming better human beings because of it. We recommend encouragement of an environment where the feelings of the father are allowed to be expressed without censure and where he is encouraged to participate and show his concern during labor and birth. At the same time we realize that the presence of a father in the delivery room may be controversial and that medical personnel have expressed their opinions on this practice, both pro and con. It is difficult for anyone to accept change when one approach has been working apparently well for a long time.

But we offer a challenge: We believe that parents should be given the option to decide for themselves whether they want to share the birth experience; following the dictates of a hospital denies them this freedom of choice. However, we recognize that some men choose nonparticipation, and we support them also because their decision reflects their needs. Since the first principle is to allow the couple to make the choice about whether to be together in labor and birth, fathers should never be forced to participate against their will or made to feel guilty if they choose not to participate. Because we also recognize that some women do not want the father present at the birth, feeling that the birth process exposes them in a way in which they do not wish to be seen, we respect those wishes also. Nevertheless, we encourage these decisions to be made ahead of the day of birth by discussions with the father, mother, physician, nurse, and family—not left to a last-minute rush decision.

In the past fifteen years it has been our observation that most participating fathers think of their help in labor and birth as essential to their experience as expectant fathers. It is a satisfying and moving experience for a well-prepared father to be at the side of the mother when their baby is born, and he can be a tremendous help to her as well.

It is our sincere wish that all those who read and experience this book will finally close it with a new understanding of fathers—of who they are and who they might be. Leo Tolstoy once said: "Everybody thinks of changing humanity and nobody thinks of changing himself." What a better place to change than with the beginning?

Celeste R. Phillips
Joseph T. Anzalone

We would like to take this opportunity to thank all the fathers and the mothers who shared with us their feelings at the births of their children; and the hundreds of couples who, through the years, have taught us so much. Also, we sincerely appreciate the typing skills of our friend, Elsie Ciapponi, and the dedicated searching and communication with fathers done by Karen Nagel.

Joseph Anzalone and Celeste Phillips

My special thanks also go to my daughter, Catherine, and my son, Duncan, who did the necessary work around the house when I was writing, and to Roger, my devoted husband, whose patience and encouragement made this all possible.

Celeste Phillips

Contents

UNIT I   The prospective father, 1

UNIT II   The physician's viewpoint, 18
          Joseph T. Anzalone

UNIT III Family-centered care, 37

UNIT IV   Birth experiences, 58

UNIT V   Birth in retrospect, 120

          Epilogue, 145

          Glossary, 147

UNIT I

The prospective father

CULTURAL INFLUENCES ON FATHER'S ROLE

The family is the oldest human institution. It is society's most basic unit, surviving throughout the centuries because it serves vital human needs. Although there may be different styles of family living and different ways of relating the family to the society, the family in some form will continue to exist as long as the human race exists on earth.[30]

In a family each member assumes a role to which the culture dictates behavioral expectations, both overt and covert, and the way in which the family members see each role may vary greatly from culture to culture.[38] As the society changes, role expectations change with each new generation adapting to the changing times, although always within socially imposed limitations. Throughout history, societies have always defined the limits with which people may change their behavior without violating the unwritten rules of the culture.

Although birth is an event that is treated with importance in most cultures, attitudes toward the birth process vary considerably among different societies. For some cultures birth is a social event, with open attendance by all friends and family; for other cultures birth is conducted in secrecy.

Even though the father's role in labor and birth varied from one primitive culture to another and was often stylized and ritualistic, he

1

usually assumed an active supporting role and assisted when needed. One of the rituals that expectant fathers have practiced in primitive cultures is the ritual "couvade" in which the expectant father actually goes to bed and pretends to be in labor at or about the time the woman is laboring. He may moan and groan and seem to be experiencing the same sensations which women have described as the birth experience in that culture. The anthropologist Sir Edward Tylor named this ritual couvade in 1865 by taking the term from the French verb *couver,* to brood or hatch.[44] Some anthropologists explain couvade as an attempt by the father to declare his importance in parenting, whereas others believe the ritual permits the father to express his conflicting emotions regarding the birth and his fatherhood. Whatever the reason for the ritual, there is no doubt that it has allowed primitive fathers to be actively involved in birth for centuries, since it would be difficult to ignore the father's presence as he moans and groans on his birthing bed.

Because many cultures did not remain primitive and most Western societies became highly complex, their childbirth rituals became more complex also. It became standard in most Western cultures for the "wise women" of the community to take over as birth attendants and later gain skills and reputations as midwives. Then as these societies became even more complex and medical science developed, childbirth was gradually given over to the medical profession. In each one of these successive steps, the father's role at birth was less clearly defined, until he was finally excluded from the labor and birth process. It is interesting to note that the father's removal from the birth process closely parallels his diminished role in early child rearing in Western cultures.[37]

FATHER'S ROLE IN CHILD REARING
Nineteenth century

In Western society the ideal nineteenth-century father was self-reliant, strong, resolute, courageous, honest, hard working, and capable of filling the traditional role of breadwinner.[14] The father's home was his castle, and he was both respected and feared by his children; in many ways he functioned as absolute ruler. Society was structured so that the father often worked as a skilled tradesman, farmer, or shopkeeper at or near his home; consequently, it was easy for the children to identify with him and his role. If the father operated a tinsmith shop at the back of the yard, the children could watch him work and conduct business so that they knew who he was and what skills he had, and thus they understood his importance to them.

Although all actual physical aspects of child care may have been left

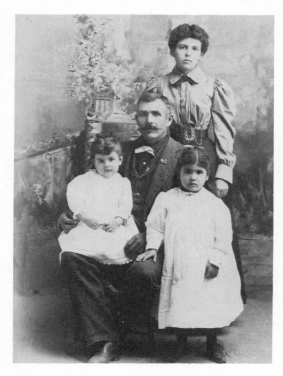

Late nineteenth-century family.

to the mother, the father often determined what was to become of the lives of both mother and children, ruling the roost often with an iron hand.[38]

Childbirth was accepted as part of the life cycle, usually occurring at home with the assistance of a midwife, woman relative, or the family physician. The father could choose to wait in the house with male friends or relatives or to go about his work at or near the home until the baby's arrival was announced. At times he would be needed to boil water, carry in firewood, build a fire, or generally help prepare the birth environment. But whether or not he was active in physical preparations, the father was proudly although distantly interested in the pregnancy and birth.

Twentieth century

The father's absolute power in the home began to decline as social reforms swept over society in the United States in the early 1900s and

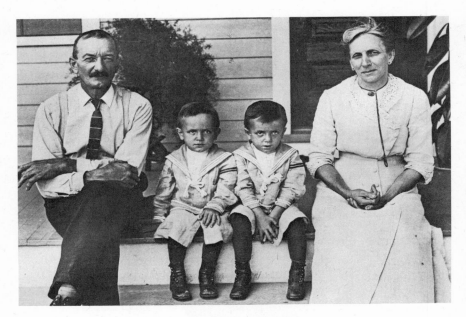

Family in the early 1900s.

women's rights became an issue. Trade unions and democratic developments proliferated, and mothers and children began to make demands for democracy in the home, speaking openly of partnership in the home and of equality of the sexes. As the voices for equality became louder, society unseated the father, declaring that he had held the power too long. Unfortunately, the attack was so strong that in denying paternalism it also denied fatherhood.[5]

Because industrialization and urbanization were occurring in Western society at the same time, a father often found himself now working a long distance from the home and working long hours, often from sunrise to sunset. As the father spent more and more time away from home, many traditional functions of the father were inherited by the mother. It became necessary for the father to delegate his place in early child rearing to the mother, and thus the mother's domain became the home and children whereas the father's domain became his world of work. Increasingly, men were measured not by what they did or how well they did it but by how much money they earned. A father became valuable in the society when he became a "good provider."[19] When World War II brought women into the work force, where many stayed, the cultural sex roles in the United States changed rapidly with the trend to equality of the sexes eliminating any authority the father had left.

Also, as society became more complex and industrialized, the role of institutions in people's lives became more important. The setting for childbirth began to move into hospitals for those who could afford them, and now instead of waiting in his parlor or his shop for his child to be born, the father found himself waiting in a hospital's Father's Waiting Room, designed just for him. Large cities were building beautiful modern women's hospitals with well-equipped modern obstetrical units, where the mystique surrounding birth could isolate the father even more.[14]

SEX ROLES

As this short historical review has pointed out, the sex roles of men and women in the United States were tightly drawn and rigid. Since many men in our society have been raised in an atmosphere of antifathering, most people think that it is unmanly for a man to overtly and spontaneously express his emotions, break down in tears, and generally be openly emotional. Most people react with embarrassment or disgust at a man's inability to "control himself."[17]

According to the cultural norm a woman should be soft, passive, tender, loving, and able to respond emotionally. To be a woman is to be nurturing—that is, motherly. A man, on the other hand, has had to repress his feelings of tenderness and gentleness, causing him to deemphasize his role as father, thus making fatherhood a social obligation[23] and motherhood a biological obligation. These strict sex-role definitions have helped to exclude men from the women's wards of our hospitals, where most childbearing occurs in our society. In contemporary culture childbirth is often surrounded by mystery, behind the hospital doors

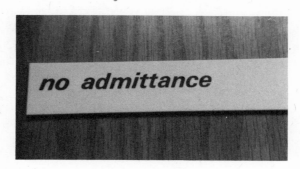

Childbirth surrounded by mystery.

marked No Admittance. Furthermore, being present at birth is an event often reserved only for medical personnel.

The denial of permission to men to become emotionally committed to childbearing and child rearing has made many fathers believe that they are unnecessary participants in pregnancy and birth.[5] At the same time it is ironical that in reality the role of the father is tremendously important for the mental health of the family. Study after study indicates that emotional disturbances in children can be traced to the detachment or lack of involvement of a father with his children.[38] There is evidence that early paternal deprivation has a significant influence on a child's personality development.[34]

It is also clear that in the relationship between a man and a woman, the way in which a woman feels about her mate is extremely important. A woman is not free to truly express her motherliness until the father of her child can express his fatherliness.[38]

Since the early 1950s, large numbers of fathers and fathers-to-be began to wonder if there may not be a better way to be introduced to fatherhood, and thus they began attending classes on marriage and the family.[14] As men have become more involved in pregnancy and birth, women have been finding a new freedom. Sharing in childbearing and

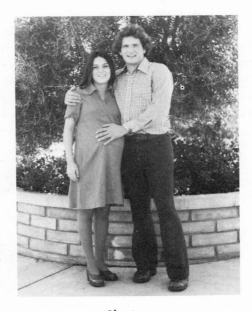

Sharing.

child rearing is helping to redefine sex roles for women, too, and as more and more fathers are actively involved in fatherhood, no longer is a woman's destiny chained to her biology.

MEANING AND EFFECT OF PREGNANCY ON FATHERS

Women undergo an extensive social preparation for motherhood that includes baby showers, maternity clothes, coffee klatches to discuss babies, magazine and newspaper articles on mothers and babies, and numerous well-wishing, advice-giving friends, neighbors, co-workers, and relatives. Men do not undergo an extensive social preparation for fatherhood, even though pregnancy is a crucial time for them also.[5]

The reactions of men to fatherhood are many and diverse, and although many expectant fathers have a so-called normal joyful reaction to impending fatherhood, some may react with depression, fear, anger, or jealousy.[39] How a man reacts to impending fatherhood may depend on his childhood memories of his own father, his mother's pregnancies, and his own childhood.[22] A man's relationship with the mother of his child before the pregnancy will also influence his reaction to fatherhood. All these factors influence the way in which he views his male sex role.

Extensive experience with expectant fathers who have actively involved themselves in pregnancy and birth indicates that most men go through stages in becoming a father. The first introduction to fatherhood comes with the confirmation of the diagnosis of pregnancy, to which men often react with unclear feelings of what being a father means to them. The first perceptible movements of the fetus in the uterus create in most men a profound and moving realization that the child is real, with most fathers recalling the time when they first "felt the baby move." During the second half of pregnancy, when the woman's pregnancy becomes physically obvious, men begin to think seriously about being a father, noticing babies and other pregnant women, sometimes for the first time. In summary, the pregnancy confirmation, fetal movement, and the growing uterus are important events for men to experience as they adapt to fatherhood—especially for the first time.[36]

During pregnancy a man must deal with the role change of his wife/lover to mother at the same time that he is becoming a father. In addition, he may be further confused by the woman's beginning to evaluate him in terms of what kind of a father he will be, even though he may be unsure and feeling strongly dependent himself.[49]

Pregnancy is no cure for a failing relationship or a failing marriage; instead it can be a real testing ground for a man-woman relationship in addition to the training ground for parenthood. The old adage, "All they need is a baby to help them grow up and solve their problems," has no origin in fact at all.

Many studies support the theory that pregnancy is a crisis time for men as well as women. In a study of expectant fathers by Liebenberg,[27] many men expressed pleasure that the pregnancy was confirmed but anxiety about whether they could handle the emotional and financial responsibilities. In writing about the "Crisis of Becoming a Father," Arnstein[4] reported arrest rates for sex offenses, which were apparently significantly higher for expectant fathers. Wainright,[45] in a review of 10 case histories, found fatherhood to be a precipitation factor in mental illness in men who had personality matrixes that were vulnerable.

It is not unusual for some men to acquire unintentionally the symptoms presented by the pregnant woman and feel nauseated during the first trimester or feel stomach cramps when the woman is in labor. Leibenberg[27] reported that 65% of 64 first-time expectant fathers reported "pregnancy symptoms," including fatigue in the first trimester and nausea, backache, headache, vomiting, and peptic ulcer. One theory which has been proposed to explain this phenomenon is that it represents an anxiety state precipitated by concern over the pregnancy.[41] Other theories include (1) unconscious expression of the father's pregnant emotional state,[2] (2) envy of pregnancy,[27] and (3) unconscious resistance to fatherhood.[17]

McHall and Glasener[29] interviewed 15 first-time fathers on the second or third day after their baby's birth and found that the financial responsibilities of having a new baby created concern for two thirds of these fathers. Wapner[46] also found that the issue of being responsible and providing for a young family was a major concern of 128 first-time expectant fathers.

LeMasters[26] studied 46 urban, middle-class couples through pregnancy and childbirth and reported that 38 of them experienced extensive or severe crisis in adjusting to their first child. Most couples had romanticized the parent role and were not prepared for the reality of dirty diapers, 2 A.M. feedings, vomiting formula, crying, and other responsibilities.

Although there is much evidence to support the theory that pregnancy is a crisis time for fathers, psychologically healthy men can and do handle pregnancy and birth without major problems. They simply find ways of coping. Many men react to pregnancy by working unusually hard, particularly during the first months, often expressing a wish to get ahead and to save for purchases, physician bills, and the baby. Whether this is the true reason for such frantic energy is debatable, since they may be using extra-hard work as a way to relieve anxiety and restlessness.

There is no doubt about it—pregnancy is an adjustment period for expectant fathers, and it may even be as much of an adjustment period for them as it is for expectant mothers. [29]

The labor and birth itself, as the culmination of pregnancy and the beginning of the relationship between father and child, can have a significant influence on the father. Many physicians who are experienced with participating fathers believe that the more interest the husband is encouraged to take in pregnancy the more likely he is to welcome the opportunity of being with his wife in labor. [41]

FATHER'S PARTICIPATION IN LABOR AND BIRTH

In today's mother-centered culture, however, it is only relatively recently that fathers have begun to be welcomed at the hospital delivery.

When women began to be hospitalized for childbirth, it seems that the father lost his role. In an effort to reduce infections in the delivery unit, all visitors were excluded. Unfortunately, the term "visitor" included anyone *but* hospital personnel, and thus the father was viewed as a possible source of contamination and was relegated to a waiting room. Maternal and infant morbidity and mortality statistics improved, but the separation of the father from the mother during labor and birth caused a change in attitude toward the birth itself. Childbirth became a medical procedure—something that was done to the woman not something that was done by her.

However, many women were beginning to believe that something was missing in this stainless steel, aseptic environment. As they were left to labor, separated from family and friends, they found that busy nurses could not spend hour after hour with one laboring woman; consequently, she was often left to labor alone, anxious and apprehensive in a narrow hospital labor bed.. Drugs that promised relief from pain and memory of pain fulfilled their promise but often left an empty feeling—a feeling of "What happened? Where am I?" "Am I really a mother now?" "Is that stranger my baby?"

PREPARATION FOR CHILDBIRTH

In 1932 Grantly Dick-Read, an obstetrician, began to teach and speak on the subject of natural childbirth and wrote *Childbirth Without Fear*. [11] Read made a great contribution to childbirth by explaining that this event could be an exhilarating experience for a woman and by demonstrating a way in which this could be achieved. Prior to the publication of Read's book, there was little reference made in obstetrical texts about the influence of emotions on labor. The women who had been searching for a better way of giving birth eagerly read his theory on the "fear-tension-pain syndrome," which explained that the discomforts of normal labor can be caused by the effects of fear and tension. Women began preparing themselves, using Read's methods, and found that their pain was relieved and birth was a rewarding experience again.

New methods of controlling pain in childbirth were introduced in the late 1940s in the Soviet Union, utilizing Pavlovian psychology and coining the term "psychoprophylaxis" in obstetrics. In 1952 Fernand Lamaze visited Russia and brought the methods of psychoprophylaxis to Paris. Women trained in this method are taught to understand the physiological and psychological aspects of pregnancy, labor, and birth and to learn body conditioning and control through exercises and breathing techniques. Team work during labor and birth is stressed, and the father becomes the logical team member because he is readily available in the home for breathing practice and is emotionally involved in experiencing a "good" pregnancy and birth. Some women found the Read methods too spiritual and ethereal for them and welcomed the more scientific approach of psychoprophylaxis.

Since 1950 there have been many other philosophies of prepared childbirth that did not depend on drugs for relief of pain. However, in addition to giving the woman control over her own body, an important change that was implemented as a result of all of these methods was to bring the father back to the labor and delivery rooms. In many instances nurses welcomed the father because the labor experience improved for all involved when he functioned as a team member, and as women had their basic need for a supporting presence fulfilled, they told other women of their shared births. When men were not separated from their wives in labor and birth, their anxiety was lessened and they talked openly about their improved experiences.

Some hospitals responded to these prepared couples by opening the delivery rooms to the fathers. Other hospitals responded by closing the delivery room doors even more tightly. In some areas of the United States men handcuffed themselves to their wives in labor so that they could not be separated.

LEGISLATION RELATIVE TO FATHER PARTICIPATION

On October 23, 1964, the California State Board of Health formally adopted a new rule permitting hospitals to allow expectant fathers to be present at the birth of their children. Soon after, in the summer of 1967, the Illinois Hospital Licensing Act was revised to allow husbands in the delivery room with the consent of attending physician and expectant mother.[40]

Nevertheless, regulations concerning father participation in labor and birth still vary from state to state. Many state departments of health have no formal written policies or regulations regarding fathers in delivery rooms, whereas some states have removed such restrictions. Even in states where restrictions are removed, some hospitals define father to mean husband and will only include legally married men in birth participation. On March 25, 1974, the Montana Supreme Court ruled in favor of the hospital in a father-access case, thus preventing fathers in the delivery room in that hospital. Active support to couples attempting to challenge such decisions is offered by childbirth education groups, such as the International Childbirth Education Association (ICEA), and other international federations of groups and individuals interested in family-centered maternity and infant care.[36]

Some medical personnel who discourage the presence of fathers in delivery rooms argue that they would increase the risk of infections, encourage malpractice suits, cause confusion if they get in the way or faint, and make hospital personnel uncomfortable. Some argue that if emergency resuscitation is needed, fathers may witness medical procedures that might frighten them.[40]

It was not until 1974 that the American College of Obstetricians and Gynecologists endorsed the concept of the husband or "other companion" remaining with the woman in labor, with the provision that adequate obstetrical facilities were present and that the attending physician agreed.[1]

STUDIES SUPPORTING FATHER PARTICIPATION

Data from thousands of births at which fathers were present have been compiled, and all these studies and surveys refute the objections against father participation in childbirth.

In more than 45,000 husband-attended births surveyed by the ICEA in 1965, there was not one infection or one malpractice suit traceable to the father's presence in the delivery room.[21]

In 1972 a questionnaire to gather data on father participation at birth was sent to all United States hospitals that listed a maternity service. Of 5,403 questionnaires sent, 1,248 were returned, listing 320,230 births. Fathers were admitted to the delivery room in only 27.2% of these births (87,208). In addition, the survey found no puerperal infections traceable to father participation at birth. Two respondents stated that they had malpractice suits or threats traceable to father participation—one if the hospital refused to allow the father in the delivery room and the other by the child's father for "mishandling the infant."[13]

Robert Bradley, an obstetrician and proponent of husband-coached childbirth, reports that, having attended over 13,000 natural births for over twenty-six years, the husband should be the one in constant attendance. He writes that the only "handicap" he has found in these births is the excess of enthusiasm of the parents afterward.[6]

Wonnell,[48] at the Wilmington Medical Center, Delaware, reported that in over 6,000 births that were attended by fathers who had taken part in a childbirth preparation program, not one father fainted. In fact, the fathers often gained a respect for the obstetrician when they were present at an obstetrical emergency.

From 1952 to 1963, 11,305 fathers participated in their baby's birth at the Mason Clinic in Seattle. The infection rate was not increased, and the presence of the father caused no problems.[33]

In Massachusetts, in eighteen months of father participation at birth, there were no fainting fathers.[15]

In a study of 1,000 consecutive births under a training-for-childbirth program at Yale–New Haven Hospital (January 1, 1949, to March 31, 1950), positive comments on the program were reported by all participants.[43]

John Miller, a former Chief of Obstetrics at French Hospital, San Francisco, has written eloquently of having participated in or observed thousands of husband-attended births and of finding them "joyous."[31]

Nevertheless, all the joyous reports of shared births and surveys reporting thousands of safely attended births have still not resulted in the opening of all delivery room doors to fathers who choose and ask to enter. Change is as slow and painful as it is inevitable. Men and women have been known to acquire feelings of territoriality, just as animals do, staking out their own ground and defending it as an exclusive preserve. Birth in the hospital occurs in the territory of medicine. It is extremely difficult to open up the territory in which one feels so secure.[3] It will not happen quickly, but happen it must.

BENEFITS OF FATHER PARTICIPATION

From the fathers who are participating and speaking out, the data are being compiled to support their new role in which they receive a vital introduction to fatherhood. Studies have shown that the father's presence in the labor room results in a decreased need for analgesia[12] and that his supportive presence can enable labor to be a valuable interpersonal experience for the couple.[16] Evaluations from 145 women who participated in a prepared childbirth program stressed the usefulness of having their husband present during labor and birth to aid them in control. These women believed that having a familiar person with them in labor helped to combat their sense of isolation or alienation.[47]

In investigating the role of husbands in labor and birth, Tanzer[42] compared groups in which the husband was present or absent at birth. The results of this study indicate that the wives experienced a positive and highly desirable effect when their husbands were present during birth. All women who reported a rapturous or peak experience during birth had their husbands present in the delivery room.

A survey published in *American Baby,* June, 1972, reported that from 2,796 responses, 80% of both husbands and wives were positive about the childbirth experience. Not all couples thought that the husband was useful in the delivery room, but they were more positive about his presence and assistance during labor. The conclusions drawn were that "something significant is happening," and there is a need to explore attitudes about childbearing in this country further.[8]

Cogan and Henneborn[9] studied two groups of couples, all enrolled in childbirth education classes. In one group fathers attended labor and birth, and in the second group fathers attended only the first stage of labor. In the total participation group the women reported less pain, received less medication, and reported more positive feelings about the total birth experience than in the partial participation group.

Cronenwett and Newmark[10] questioned 158 fathers who expressed their feelings about their infants and wives during labor and birth. Fathers with preparation and/or those who attended the birth rated their overall experiences during childbirth significantly more positively than the fathers who did not have these experiences. According to this study, even without preparation, attendance at the birth positively influenced the couple's relationship.

A doctoral dissertation by Hott[20] showed that there was a similarity of self-concept and concept of their wives among participating and non-participating fathers in labor and birth. This study would seem to dispel the theories often put forth by professionals and lay people that men who want to be present at birth are morbidly curious, or zealots of "natural childbirth," or are wanting to experience an ego trip.

In a moving report on a personal tragedy, the birth and death of their newborn, a woman writes of the comforting presence of her husband in the delivery room and how relieved she was that she never had to explain the death to her husband because he was there with her all the time.[7]

Over and over again these studies demonstrate that the father's presence in the labor and delivery rooms is helpful in reducing the woman's feeling of loneliness and rejection. There seem to be threads running throughout these studies of a feeling of sharing an experience and deepening a relationship. There also seems to be an implication that a higher level of consciousness for men may be developing—that participating and sharing in labor and birth affirms the paternal role implicitly, in a tangible and real way, as the father recognizes the baby as his.

BONDING—PATERNAL-INFANT ATTACHMENT

Finally, in our discussion of father participation in childbirth, we must consider the subject of bonding. Marshall Klaus and his colleagues have been actively studying whether human mothers have a "sensitive period" immediately after birth, as has been reported among animal mothers. In many animals, if the mother and baby are separated immediately after birth, the mother will reject her young when they are reunited—even after a separation of only 1 or 2 hours. Conversely, if the animal mother and baby are together in the first few days, then separated and reunited, the mother quickly accepts the baby. Klaus and his colleagues [24] have also found that human mothers who have close contact with their babies immediately after birth are more responsive and sensitive to their babies' needs. This phenomenon is termed "bonding," or "imprinting"—the baby is imprinted on the mother's consciousness.

Imprinting may also be necessary to the development of fatherliness. Findings from animal research seem to indicate that early contact between a father and his infant seems to encourage paternal behavior. Laboratory research with rats shows that male mice and rats develop maternal-like behavior when exposed to infant mice and rats. Research with primates has shown that after 15 minutes in contact with 1-month-old rhesus monkeys, 8 out of 15 preadolescent male monkeys exhibited maternal behavior. Redican and Mitchell have had adult male rhesus monkeys in individual laboratory cages actually rear baby monkeys in the absence of their mothers. This animal research seems to indicate that newborns have a strong impact on males in many species and that when the male's exposure to the newborn was increased, they became more involved in newborn care. [28]

Can we speculate from this animal research that men who are exposed to their own newborns will become more involved in child rearing also? There is an interesting study by Greenberg and Morris [18] that seems to give some credence to this speculation. They studied first-time fathers in two groups of 15 individuals. The first group had contact with the newborn in the delivery room, whereas the second group had contact with the newborn after the birth; in each case in the second group the baby was shown to them by a nurse. Overwhelmingly, fathers who were present at their baby's birth believed that they could always distinguish their baby from other babies by how he looked. The fathers who were not present at birth thought that they could do this only some of the time.[18]

A study by Parke[35] to determine to what extent fathers interact with 2- to 4-day-old infants in hospital situations showed that the father clearly played a more active role in infant contact than culture in the United States has acknowledged.

Data from Stockholm indicated that fathers who spent 30 minutes with their nude newborn later spent more hours playing with the baby at 3 months of age than fathers who had not been granted that 30 minutes of contact.[25]

This growing body of evidence on the importance of infant-parent bonding tends to support the practice of preparing couples for childbirth. Furthermore, it seems crucial that in a society such as that in the United States, where opportunities for individual growth and development are unlimited, men should have the right to experience fatherhood to the fullest.

REFERENCES

1. American College of Obstetricians and Gynecologists. Standards for Obstetric-Gynecologic Services, Chicago, 1974, The College.
2. Antle, K.: Psychologic involvement in pregnancy by expectant fathers, Journal of Obstetric, Gynecologic and Neonatal Nursing, pp. 40-42, July/Aug., 1975.
3. Ardrey, R.: The territorial imperative, New York, 1966, Dell Publishing Co., Inc.
4. Arnstein, H.: The crisis of becoming a father, Sexual Behavior pp. 42-47, April, 1972.
5. Biller, H. B., and Meredith, D.: Father power, New York, 1975, David McKay Co., Inc.
6. Bradley, R. A.: Husband-coached childbirth, New York, 1974, Harper & Row, Publishers.
7. Breuer, J.: Sharing a Tragedy, American Journal of Nursing **76:**758-759, 1976.
8. Childbearing is a family affair, ICEA News **12:**9, Summer, 1973.
9. Cogan, R., and Henneborn, W. J.: The effect of husband participation on reported pain and probability of medication during labor and birth, Journal of Psychosomatic Research **19:**215-222, 1975.
10. Cronenwett, L. R., and Newmark, L. L.: Fathers' responses to childbirth, Nursing Research **23:**210-217, 1974.
11. Dick-Read, G.: Childbirth without fear, New York, 1953, Harper & Row, Publishers.
12. Engel, E. L.: Family centered maternity care, Obstetrics/Gynecology Digest, pp. 25-32, Nov., 1964.
13. Ernst, S., editor: Father participation guide, Rochester, N.Y., May, 1975, International Childbirth Education Association, Inc.
14. Filene, P. G.: Him/her/self: sex, roles in modern America, New York, 1975, Harcourt Brace Jovanovich, Inc.

15. Gleming, G.: Delivering a happy father, American Journal of Nursing **72**:949, 1972.
16. Goetsch, C.: Fathers in the delivery room—helpful and supportive, Hospital Topics **44**:104, Jan., 1966.
17. Goldberg, H.: The hazards of being male, Plainview, N.Y., 1976, Nash Publishing Corp.
18. Greenberg, M., and Morris, N.: Engrossment: the newborn's impact upon the father, American Journal of Orthopsychiatry **44**:520-531, 1974.
19. Hines, J.: Father, the forgotten man, Nursing Forum **10**:177-200, 1971.
20. Hott, J. R.: An investigation of the relationship between psychoprophylaxis in childbirth and changes in self-concept of the participant husband and his concept of his wife, Ph.D. dissertation, New York University, New York, 1972.
21. International Childbirth Education Association: Husbands in the delivery room: recommendations to hospital administrators and physicians on the desirability and safety of the practice, Rochester, N.Y., April, 1965, The Association.
22. Jarvis, W.: Some effects of pregnancy and childbirth on men, Journal of the American Psychoanalytic Association **10**:689-700, 1969.
23. Josselyn, I.: Cultural forces, motherliness and fatherliness, Children, pp. 264-271, May/June, 1964.
24. Klaus, M. H., Jerauld, R., Kreger, N. C., McAlpine, W., Steffa, M., and Kenrell, J. H.: Maternal attachment: importance of the first post-partum days, New England Journal of Medicine **286**:460-463, 1972.
25. Klaus, M. H.: Presentation at De Anza College, Cupertino, Calif., May 14, 1976.
26. LeMasters, E.: Parenthood as crisis. In Parad, H. J., editor: Crisis intervention: selected readings, New York, 1971, Family Service Association of America.
27. Liebenberg, B.: Expectant fathers, Child and Family **8**:264-267, Summer, 1969.
28. Lynn, D. B.: The father: his role in child development, Monterey, Calif., 1974, Brooks/Cole Publishing Co.
29. McHall, L. K., and Glasener, J.: Current practice in obstetric and gynecologic nursing, vol. 1, St. Louis, 1976, The C. V. Mosby Co.
30. Mead, M., and Heyman, K.: Family, New York, 1965, The Macmillan Co.
31. Miller, J. S.: Return the joy of home delivery with fathers in the delivery room, Hospital Topics, 105-109, Jan., 1966.
32. Montana Supreme Court Appeal, ICEA News **13**:1, 14, Summer, 1974.
33. Moore, D. C., and Bridenbaugh, L. D.: Physician, anesthesia, regional block and father participation: the ultimate in care of vaginal delivery, Western Journal of Surgery, Obstetrics and Gynecology **72**:37-44, Jan.-Feb., 1964.
34. Nash, J.: The father in contemporary culture and current psychological literature, Child Development **36**:261-297, March, 1965.
35. Parke, R. D.: Father-infant interaction. In Klaus, M. H., Leger, T., and Trause, M. A., editors: Maternal attachment and mothering disorders, a round table, Johnson & Johnson Baby Products Co., Sausalito, Calif., Oct. 18-19, 1974.
36. Phillips, C.: Interviews with fathers, 1974-1976, (unpublished) manuscript.
37. Richardson, S. A., and Allan F.: Childbearing—its social and psychological aspects, Baltimore, 1967, The Williams & Wilkins Co., pp. 164-169, 172, 190.
38. Robischon, P., and Scott, D.: Role theory and its application in family nursing, Nursing Outlook **17**:52-57, July, 1969.
39. Schaefer, G. and Zisowitz, M. L.: The expectant father, New York, 1964, Simon & Schuster, Inc., Publishers.
40. Shu, C.: Husband-father in delivery room, Hospitals **47**:90 passim, Sept. 16, 1973.
41. Stallworthy, J.: Management of the hospital confinement. In Howells, J. G., editor: Modern perspectives in psycho-obstetrics, New York, 1972, Brunner/Mazel, Inc.
42. Tanzer, D. S.: The psychology of pregnancy and childbirth: an investigation of natural childbirth, unpublished Ph.D. dissertation, Brandeis University, Waltham, Mass., 1967, University Microfilms.

43. Thoms, H., and Karloosky, E.: 2000 Deliveries under training for childbirth program, American Journal of Obstetrics and Gynecology 68:279-284, 1954.
44. Trethowan, W. H.: The couvade syndrome. In Howells, J. G., editor: Modern perspectives in psycho-obstetrics, New York, 1972, Brunner/Mazel, Inc.
45. Wainright, W. H.: Fatherhood as a precipitant of mental illness, American Journal of Psychiatry 123:44, 1966.
46. Wapner, J.: The attitudes, feelings and behaviors of expectant fathers attending Lamaze classes, Birth and the Family Journal 3:5-13, Spring, 1976.
47. Willmuth, L. R.: Prepared childbirth and the concept of control, Journal of Obstetric, Gynecologic, and Neonatal Nursing, pp. 38-41, Sept./Oct., 1975.
48. Wonnell, E. B.: The education of the expectant father for childbirth, Nursing Clinics of North America 6:591-603, 1971.
49. Woods, N. F.: Human sexuality in health and illness, St. Louis, 1975, The C. V. Mosby Co.

ADDITIONAL READINGS

Bancroft, A. V.: Pregnancy and the counterculture, Nursing Clinics of North America 8:67-76, March, 1973.
Bartemeier, L.: The contribution of the father to the mental health of the family, American Journal of Psychiatry 110:278, 1953.
Benson, L.: Fatherhood, a sociological perspective, New York, 1968, Random House, Inc.
Chabon, I.: Awake and aware: participating in childbirth through psychoprophylaxis, New York, 1966, Delacorte Press.
Chiota, B. J., Goolkasian, P., and Ladeqig, P.: Effects of separation from spouse on pregnancy, labor and delivery, and the postpartum period, Journal of Obstetric, Gynecologic and Neonatal Nursing, pp. 21-23, Jan./Feb., 1976.
Clausen, J. P., Flook, M. H., Ford, B., Green, M. M., and Popiel, E. S.: Maternity nursing today, New York, 1973, McGraw-Hill Book Co.
Cogan, R.: Comfort during prepared childbirth as a function of parity, reported by four classes of participant observers, Journal of Psychosomatic Research 19:33-37, 1975.
Cogan, R., and Klopper, F.: The delivery of childbirth reports: an analysis of sample bias in questionnaire returns, Journal of Psychosomatic Research 19:39-42, 1975.
Eiderson, B. T., et al.: Alternatives in child rearing in the 1970's, American Journal of Orthopsychiatry, 43:720-731, 1973.
Gagnon, J., and Henderson, B.: Human sexuality, an age ambiguity, Social Issues Series, no. 1, Boston, 1975, Little, Brown & Co., Inc.
Genedek, T.: Insight and personality, New York, 1946, Ronald Press & Co.
Genné, W. H.: Husbands and pregnancy, St. Meinrad, Ind., 1956, Abbey Press.
Goerzen, J. L., and Chinn, P. L.: Review of maternal and child nursing, St. Louis, 1975, The C. V. Mosby Co.
Heise, J.: Toward better preparation for involved fatherhood, Journal of obstetric, Gynecologic and Neonatal Nursing, pp. 32-35, Sept., Oct., 1975.
Kitzinger, S.: Giving birth: the parents' emotions in childbirth, London, 1971, Victor Gollancz, Ltd.
Lesser, M. and Keane, V.: Nurse-patient relationships in a hospital maternity service, 1956, St. Louis, The C. V. Mosby Co.
Marquart, R. K.: Expectant fathers: what are their needs? MCN The American Journal of Maternal Child Nursing, pp. 32-36, Jan., Feb., 1976.
Reeder, S. R., Mastroianni, L. Jr., Martin, L. L., and Fitzpatrick, E.: Maternity nursing, ed. 13, Philadelphia, 1976, J. B. Lippincott Co.

UNIT II

The physician's viewpoint

Joseph T. Anzalone

Probably any father, any husband, would really like to have some idea about what the physician thinks of his being in the delivery room. In this chapter I hope to demonstrate that fathers are more than just a physical presence—they are needed and they are important.

Over the past six years I have delivered well over two thousand babies with the father present. Currently, about 95% of the births at Santa Cruz Dominican and Community Hospitals take place with the father in the delivery room. This experience has convinced me beyond any doubt that there need not be any problems with having the father present at the time of birth. In fact, I need him there.

However, I know that many physicians take a different attitude toward this concept. Some are cautious; others are openly hostile. These competent men and women have formed their views on the basis of their own unique experiences. They are sincerely concerned with the welfare of the pregnant woman. Even though my own experience has been so positive, it should not be held against that of any other practitioner who takes a different view. Contrasting viewpoints do not mean that one individual's capabilities as a physician are less than those of another physician. This is one area where it is vital to preserve the physician's freedom of practice.

With these thoughts in mind, I want to relate my experiences. I tell this in a personal way because that is how it has validity for me, since a physician is a person, too. I will describe the history, impact, and significance of the approach to birth with the father as a participant and then outline the educational program that has evolved in my practice to make all of this possible. Finally, in a hypothetical interview, I will examine some doubts that a prospective father still might have about whether, after all, he *really* wants to be there at the moment of birth.

HOW IT ALL CAME ABOUT
Consumer pressures

My involvement with obstetrics began in 1957, when I entered residency in obstetrics and gynecology after graduation from medical school. At that time no fathers were permitted in the delivery room except occasionally for a physician whose wife was giving birth. The prevailing attitude was that birth was a dangerous medical operation. It was the physician's business and nobody else's. The father was often seen as a comic figure—certainly he would be an unwanted intruder at an event that he could neither possibly understand nor appreciate. In fact, not even the mother was there because she was under anesthesia. Birth was strictly a medical event.

After several years of private obstetrical practice, when the "natural childbirth movement" began in mid-1966 in my area of the United States, it was somewhat frightening to me. I believed at the time that the father was going to be just an observer—an untrained observer who would be critical of what I was doing. He would be questioning and suspicious because he would know nothing about medicine and the problems I might encounter or the procedures I might use. He would not understand why in certain instances forceps might be necessary, and he would be upset if he saw any blood. I believed that my privacy was being invaded.

Classes started on Wednesday nights at the YWCA for women who were contemplating natural childbirth. Each woman was given ten or fifteen questions that she should ask her physician—me. So Thursday morning was chaotic in the office because every woman would come in with the same list of questions, which could not really be answered with a simple "yes" or "no." They would include questions such as "Will I need an anesthetic?" or "Will I have an episiotomy?" I could feel a sense of antagonism and even hostility as they asked the questions.

By the end of the day I had heard the same list of questions so many times that I often knew the questions better than the patients. I thought that the childbirth education instructors were better able to discuss these questions and feelings, and so my own classes were started.

There are good reasons for medical conservatism, but in this case it was the public that proved to be right in forcing a reluctant physician into progress. I found to my surprise that the women who were educated in these classes had easier births and really coped much better, requiring less time, less effort, less medication, and certainly less anesthesia.

Medicine goes through phases

Of course, so-called "natural childbirth" with the father present is not a new phenomenon. There is a pendulum effect in medicine—it goes through different phases. There was a time when all babies were born at home, and the husband must have participated to a considerable extent in those births because sometimes there was nobody else around except him. Then medicine went through a Victorian stage, when not even the physicians were allowed to examine the woman in labor. Only the nurse-midwives examined her and then reported the woman's progress to the physician, who often was in the next room. The current phase of medicine, in which fathers are present during childbirth is perhaps the best of all. It may well last the longest because there is a trend in society toward increased consumer participation and responsibility. People today want to understand and be involved in their health care. Medical terminology is a whole different language. In the old days the family physician used to give conditions names that people could understand. For example, "walking pneumonia" was pneumonia that moved from one lung to the other. The people could relate to that term and say, "Well, yeah, I have walking pneumonia; it's moving around and I can understand that."

But now, if you look at a medical dictionary, it is full of medical terms that nobody but a health professional could understand. It is a completely different language. It is just as if someone started speaking a foreign language to you and you wondered what in the world they were talking about. A gynecologist will call a white spot on the cervix "leukoplakia," which means white plaque. Well, why not just call it white plaque? A dermatologist will call scaly skin "ichthyosis." All these Latin-derived terms can really confuse people. By increasing people's understanding through education, they are better able to participate in their own care.

New meaning for the physician

To a great extent, before this new approach to childbirth began, obstetrics and gynecology had become boring—a mechanical process, the same thing over and over again. There was really no variation, and every birth was pretty much like the one before. There was no emotional gratification or reward in it for the physician. One big reason why individuals go into medicine is that it is gratifying to help people, to see a patient get well.

So I almost gave up obstetrics because it was not very fulfilling for me. Fathers in the delivery room have changed that. With the institution of classes for expectant couples, educated fathers came into the delivery room, and with that, the births really changed. They became extremely happy events. The fathers were in no way just watching or criticizing what the physician was doing because they were well-educated individuals by then—just like the physician–expectant fathers who used to be present in the delivery room occasionally.

When the mother is awake and aware and the father is there to participate and appreciate the event, I often walk out of the delivery room feeling good about the whole thing.

One word of appreciation is probably worth as much as the whole fee. When a person thanks you and says "Gee, we really enjoyed the birth and want to thank you for making it such a wonderful thing for us," that is rewarding.

Fathers improve the quality of obstetrics

When I was a resident, I moonlighted at a small hospital. It was common for a woman in labor to be given so much medication that she would remember nothing until the next day. Her husband would be downstairs in the father's room. The woman's regular physician would be at home, so I would call him and say, "Your patient has been admitted and I expect her to deliver in about 3 or 4 hours."

He would say, "Well, you deliver her and then call me." I would deliver the baby and call him and tell him this. Then he would say, "Switch me to the father's room." Through the hospital switchboard the call would be transferred to the father's room, and he would say, "Your wife just had a beautiful 9-pound boy, and in about half an hour you'll be able to go up and see the baby."

Well, the husband thought that the physician was in the hospital, yet he was home in bed. I had delivered the baby, and the woman would never know this because she had been given so much medication that she did not know who had delivered her baby. That was around 1958—so you can see how things have changed.

For a long time in the United States obstetrics was practiced at the convenience of the physician. If he had office hours, he might deliver the baby with forceps so that he could return to the office or to his home or make dinner for a dinner party. He would hasten the birth, or he might even slow it down with medication.

All that has pretty much gone by the board now. Many women are well prepared and educated and give birth with little or no medication, and their husband, or close companion, is similarly well educated and is present in the delivery room. Without question physicians practice better obstetrics now.

WHAT IT ALL MEANS

Not all physicians share my own positive feelings about having the father in the delivery room. Many have serious reservations. I believe that their fears are legitimate and honest, although in my own experience I believe that they are ill founded. Their stance does not make them less competent, less responsible, or less concerned. It would be wrong to malign a physician for concluding that the best medical practice is to have the husband excluded from participating in childbirth.

Disadvantages

Some of the most outspoken members of the "opposition" think of the delivery room as an operating room—no place for sentimentality, sightseeing, or salesmanship. These physicians believe in a strictly professional approach with "no nonsense." Their reasons for commonly excluding fathers from delivery rooms include the following:

1. It is an emotional time for the father, and his presence at birth might cause problems in his adjustment to fatherhood.
2. There is a limit to intimacy between two human beings.
3. Teaching physicians, nurses, and other hospital personnel is a continuous process, and the fathers' presence in the delivery room could interfere with this teaching process.
4. Allowing fathers in the delivery room may cause an extension of the same privilege to operating rooms and other hospital areas.
5. The presence of the father as a lay witness may be an attorney's dream and a nightmare to the defense.
6. Even if the visitor to the delivery room is dressed properly, he may be a carrier of pathogenic bacteria capable of causing infection.

Therefore, believing that it is in the best interests of the patients, "Appropriate committees have recommended to their executive medical boards that visitors to the delivery room be barred by formal statement in the by-laws of the hospital and its staff."*

*From Morton, J. H.: Fathers in the delivery room—an opposition standpoint, Hosp. Top. 4:13-14, 1967.

Passive vs. active participation

Occasionally, we have a father who is merely an observer. He has not been trained, he is not giving his wife any emotional support, but he just decided at the last minute, "I think I'll go in the delivery room and see what's going on." Although such a father may derive satisfaction from witnessing his baby's birth, he adds little or nothing to really helping his wife at the birth.

In some places today husbands put on sterile gloves and gown and deliver the baby. In uncomplicated cases anybody can deliver a baby; you can take somebody off the street and say, "OK, when the baby comes out, you catch it, don't let it fall on the floor." In most cases, I do not feel the father can perform dual roles during the birth.

He is present because he is helping his wife with both emotional and physical support. He might be supporting her back, or he might be telling her she is breathing incorrectly, or he might be counting for her while she is pushing. All of this is genuinely important and helpful—it is an *active* role for him.

"Labor" to me means "work," and it is really work to have a baby. The man and woman have to work, and they have to work together.

At one extreme the father makes love with his wife and that is all he has to do. He has done his part, and then, after nine months, she will have a baby, and somehow the baby is his because of what he did nine months before. Now, if he had made love deliberately with the thought of a baby in mind, to that extent he will feel a natural responsibility for the child. He will not think that it is something thrust on him but is a responsibility that he voluntarily assumed.

But this responsibility, which comes from his deliberate intent in making love, is limited. At every point after that, whenever he voluntarily and deliberately takes action which furthers the process of bringing the baby into being, it has a psychological effect of making him naturally and spontaneously assume more responsibility and feel more of a sense of responsibility for that child. It is more *his* child.

In summary, the father's participation in bringing the child into this world may be active or passive. If it is passive, it really is no better than watching a movie of the whole process. But active participation implies action; action leads to consequence, and deliberate action leads to responsibility for the consequence. Thus if the consequence is a child, deliberate action leading to that child results in a feeling of responsibility for the child.

By communicating, working together, and participating together in the birth, the father and mother *both* have a child. It is not just the woman who gave birth; they both worked to give birth to that child. Because they have both participated, this will be a stronger family unit. I think that is really important.

In my experience it is the childbirth training classes which make possible this meaningful, active participation on the part of the father.

PROGRESSION OF CLASSES

Health professionals must stimulate interest in prenatal education as a woman begins her pregnancy, not at the end. At the same time there is a definite progression or sequence in which classes should be taken. Sometimes a woman will come in on her first visit and ask, "Do you believe in natural childbirth?" or "Do you believe in Lamaze?" The question is premature. It is something they really should not be thinking about at that time, except perhaps to choose the physician they want. To begin the pregnancy with labor and birth is wrong; a woman has to build up to it. The interest and excitement have to peak at a certain time just as a political race or a good story. If a woman peaks too early it is downhill from there. A politician should not hit his top popularity six months before the election. If women become too excited and start off by reading the wrong books in the early part of pregnancy, they lose interest at the end. We want to take them through in such a way that they get to that point a week before they give birth instead of the beginning. In other words, the classes are not only to impart information and prepare the woman physically but also to have a psychological impact.

First visit

When a woman is seen in my office for her first prenatal visit, her education actually begins here. I explain why I am going to do a physical examination and what findings I expect. She is informed about any existing problems that should be corrected or that may have an effect later, such as a small pelvis. I usually do blood studies on the first visit, and the woman is told what will be done and the reasons for doing them. She is given an opportunity to ask questions, as many questions as she wishes, about anything she might like to know.

This is the beginning of her education. At this time I try to interest the expectant couple in attending nutrition and physiology classes.

Early pregnancy classes

We begin with two classes, one week apart, in which nutrition and hygiene are presented—information which expectant parents really should know.

For instance, the husband should be aware that early pregnancy is the time of low energy for most women. The typical woman who is two months' pregnant will sleep a lot. Most women fall asleep in the afternoon, and it is rare for a woman to last until 10 P.M. Every phase of pregnancy is geared to protect the baby. The whole biological process in humans seems to be centered around reproduction, and thus fatigue and listlessness in the early part of pregnancy allows a woman to conserve energy. This means she is saving all her fuel for the baby. If a woman is allowed to eat exactly as she did before, she will gain a lot of weight in the early part of pregnancy. This would be less desirable than gaining weight near the end, when the fetus is maturing, growing, and actually putting on most of its own weight.

The application of knowledge of early physiology with good eating habits can make early pregnancy more enjoyable. Husbands can be a great emotional support for the early hard months if they, too, know what to expect. Ignorance in these aspects can lead to much discord.

Exercise classes

After the early prenatal classes, women are encouraged to attend exercise classes weekly until the onset of labor. There are ten classes a week, allowing everyone to find a time to attend, some in the evening and some in the morning. We even have one class where mothers can bring young children so that a baby-sitter is not needed.

These classes are important both physically and emotionally. Exercise can be suggested and encouraged but not done for a person. Not only does group pressure play a part in support for exercise but here also is an excellent opportunity for women to learn appropriate specific prenatal exercises, hygiene, and physiology. This reinforces the early prenatal classes.

In my practice a certificated physical education instructor conducts these classes. She has had two children and is in excellent health. Her physical fitness is an incentive as well as a reminder that pregnancy does not have to alter a woman's body. Proper diet and exercise play a large part in emotional well-being.

An additional, although not less important, aspect is the amount of inherent positive psychological support that these women can give each other. Common problems, complaints, and joys are shared as only women, especially pregnant women, can share with each other.

This is an area where physicians, and I imagine many husbands, feel left out. This is probably rightfully so. With skillful handling and early prenatal classes, husbands can learn to encourage their wives to attend, knowing that the family will benefit. It is not that we want to discourage men—it is just that women seem to need this time alone.

In summary, exercise classes offer fitness physically and emotionally with the goal of a very pleasant and better prepared childbirth experience.

Preparation for childbirth

Toward the end of pregnancy couples begin childbirth classes. Most of our instructors are Lamaze oriented, although this is not the only technique. Fernand Lamaze was French, but the process actually originated in Russia—as a form of mind control. There is only room for a certain number of stimuli to enter an individual's mind; therefore, if you put more stimuli of one kind in, you force the stimuli of another kind out. Thus the Lamaze childbirth method is a way of giving a woman additional stimuli to distract her from the pain. This decreases the perception of pain; therefore she will feel less discomfort. If the mind dwells on severe discomfort, the muscles will tighten. When the muscles tighten, there is more discomfort, and so it goes around in a circle. As a contraction starts, one can see an unprepared person tightening and this building to a high degree of pain. If a woman has been trained in the Lamaze method or other kinds of childbirth techniques, she is "conditioned" to relax. While she is relaxing, the muscles loosen and there is less resistance to the baby's passage through the pelvis and to the labor in general. Consequently, labors are shorter and easier.

To accomplish this degree of relaxation, fear is eliminated as much as possible by explaining the labor pattern. Different breathing techniques are taught for the stages of labor. When a contraction starts, the woman breathes a certain way and concentrates on a picture or focal point. Between the visual object or stimulation and the concentration on breathing, the woman just does not have room to think about discomfort. It is like in the past, when the physician told her husband to boil water, which really was not needed for the birth but was only to occupy the husband's mind. Similarly, with the Lamaze technique a woman needs less medication. There is no room for pain stimuli to reach consciousness; they are just blocked out. Most likely the breathing technique does nothing special as far as the labor is concerned, other than distract the consciousness.

We want the prospective father to attend the childbirth preparation classes because he is the one who will coach his wife in this technique during the actual birth. In addition, the couple should be practicing regularly at home. Ideally, the couple comes to six preparatory classes during the last six weeks of pregnancy. If this is not possible, we find that even a little training is better than none. Even training given during labor itself will help.

Also during the childbirth classes, after thorough review of the process of birth, we show several films of births that have taken place in our hospital, showing the team work involved and the benefit to be gained. This helps to impart an understanding of what has been learned and the various facets about childbirth. We find that it is extremely helpful to use films as visual aids.

These childbirth classes are used to help potential mothers and fathers focus on the new life. At least one class covers the postpartum period and general newborn care.

Postpartum classes

After the woman gives birth, she may attend postpartum exercise classes. These are designed once again to bring new mothers together to share similar spaces in their life. In addition to the now routine exercises, any subject from breastfeeding to contraception is discussed.

As one can see, our educational program may last well over a year. By providing this series of classes we hope that a woman and her husband may have a more general knowledge of pregnancy, labor, birth, and the postpartum period. This helps to make pregnancy not an isolated event in one person's life but an important part of her whole life process.

Fathers and the real meaning of the class

A woman goes through many changes during her pregnancy—some obvious and expected, others less obvious and not expected. If the husband does not realize this and understand it, if he does not understand her nutritional needs and the changes that are happening to her physiologically and psychologically, the pregnancy is going to have a poor start. That is why he should be involved from the very beginning of pregnancy, and his involvement should continue throughout the process.

Then, too, a woman's pregnancy is not always a happy situation. Often the prospective father is not really excited about the idea to start off with. It may take a while for him to get used to a pregnancy. At classes other husbands and fathers are present who can share their own feelings and experiences. Many men have anxieties about their wife's being pregnant. It helps to speak about these things and to find out that others may feel the same way. It can relieve a burden of guilt and also awaken a real interest.

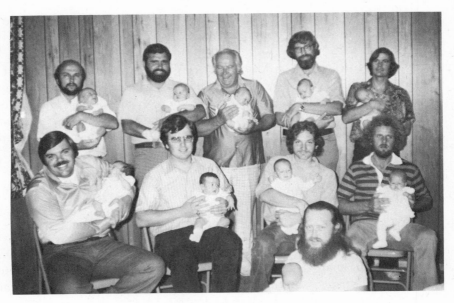

"Group psychotherapy."

If the husband is really negative about going into the delivery room, we usually encourage him to just go to the first Lamaze class. Often, that is all it takes. No husband ought to be forced into the delivery room, but he should have an opportunity to understand what it would be like, what the advantages are. Many fathers who do attend their baby's birth and have a tremendously positive experience would not even have wanted to go into the delivery room if it were not for the classes. Thus for some husbands, merely the fact that they go into the delivery room is an indication that the classes are a success.

A lot of "group psychotherapy" goes on in the classes for both the men and the women. Everyone there has questions. They all experience similar feelings and changes.

In the first Lamaze class sometimes the instructor simply goes around the room asking each person why he or she is there. By the time this has been done, one begins to realize that couples are there because they believe it is going to make the labor easier and enable a better childbirth. It is a kind of feeling that, "Well, gee whiz, I'm here because this is good; it's going to make a difference." The interest and enthusiasm is started.

If a father is going to be in the delivery room, but he does not attend the classes, his purpose and meaning in being there is lost to a great extent. He will still be able to hold the baby afterward and tell his wife what a nice baby they have, and they can spend the postpartum time together so that she is not alone, but that team work, that cooperation, that unit is lost. But when a husband comes to the classes, that couple will train together. They go to a class one night of the week, but the remainder of the week they are in training. During the week they will practice techniques that they have been taught in class. They become a team. There is no question in my mind at all that couples are brought much closer together by the husband participating in this way in the whole birth process.

Santa Cruz and the United States

We have a unique situation here in Santa Cruz. Of course, this is not the only area in the country where developments such as we have described are taking place, but it is true that Santa Cruz is unusually progressive in this respect. This is not to our own credit—it is just something which happened that way. In fact, as I explained earlier, we were forced into it here by the activities of the women's movement. The question arises—what are physicians and parents doing about this in the rest of the country?

Our whole educational program here has evolved, and is still evolving, as an adaptation to a unique set of circumstances. It developed slowly over the last ten years. We started off with just the Lamaze classes, then we added the exercise classes, and then we added the postpartum classes; now we have added the early prenatal classes. Each time we added a new segment to the program because we saw areas where we were failing to do a good job. We saw what was missing and created a class to fill the gap. Actually, the early prenatal classes were started in 1976, and they have been highly successful.

Our whole program has grown up naturally over a period of time, by response to the specific needs of this community. However, someone in another area, just starting out, may not even know where to begin.

There is a positive way of looking at this problem. The Santa Cruz program is not necessarily the ideal, but it seems to be at a stage in the development towards the ideal. Thus any other program that moves in the same direction is also advancing toward the ideal. We cannot say that our own program is completely sufficient to meet all the needs of birth training, but on the other hand, we cannot say that this is entirely necessary to provide family-centered care.

Other physicians may use our practice as a model if they wish, or they may prefer to strike out in a direction of their own, but neither they nor the prospective fathers and mothers should believe that their program is inadequate if it differs from ours. It is important for both parents and physicians to realize that each practice represents a unique situation. Each physician has had unique experiences, shaping unique attitudes and abilities, and each community also has unique expectations and needs. Physicians and parents must work together with mutual tolerance, understanding, and respect to develop the approach best suited to their own special circumstances.

At the same time I must speak briefly of three areas of concern that a physician might have when he contemplates making these changes in his own practice—time, money, and the quality of medical care.

The reader might think that this whole program, and the father's presence in the delivery room, must take up much more of my time. Actually, the reverse is true. It is saving me time in the office and it is saving me time in the delivery room, as well as making the births themselves more enjoyable. The husband in the delivery room is giving his wife emotional support throughout labor, and consequently less is required of me at that time. We, as physicians, can be freer to devote ourselves to strictly medical needs.

Time is saved also during the pregnancy. When a woman returns to our office for a visit, we ask, "Do you have any questions?" She answers, "No, I did have questions, but they were answered during exercise class. I also had some questions about nutrition, but they were all answered in the nutrition class." The classes are a big advantage to us. We can actually see more clients because we do not have to spend as much time with each woman, and yet the quality of care has improved.

It must be emphasized, however, that this does not mean that time is being saved at the client's expense. On the contrary, much more time is being spent with each woman, who is being better educated than ever before. When women were seeing only a physician and not taking classes, no one could spend the time with them that they really needed. In the classes participants spend 2 hours on nutrition alone. What physician can stop and spend 2 hours on nutrition with each client? Similarly, the time that is saved personally is still devoted to patient care. The classes free us from chores for which we were not really needed so that we can now give *each* woman *more* time for those services where a physician *is* really needed.

As for money, it is true that the staff must be paid from client fees, but because under this system we can see more people, increasing our overall volume, the total fees for obstetrical care are actually lower than those in the surrounding areas.

The hospital costs are also lower. Of course, this is also partly because we so rarely use anesthesia; thus the anesthesiologist's bill is not large and the average length of stay in the hospital is much shorter. Most women spend one night in the hospital after the birth and then go home. But regardless of the reasons, the fact is that our approach saves time and money for both the woman and the physician.

Finally, I must examine the quality of medical care that we offer under this system. The woman who has attended our classes is emotionally and physically prepared for her childbirth. The program has reduced our complication rate and also the number of what we call operative interferences in the delivery—anything from forceps to a cesarean birth. In other words, the woman will usually just give birth on her own. If we were not there, she probably would give birth just as well without us. To me, this does not mean a lessening of our role but rather a major triumph for the woman, the father, and also for obstetrics.

"BUT DOCTOR, WHAT ABOUT . . . ?"

In this obstetrical practice prospective fathers usually attend the classes, where they are introduced to the idea of being present in the delivery room before they talk with me. It would probably be better if husbands did accompany their wives on their first visit to the physician, but in our experience this usually does not happen. However, let us take "off the street" a prospective father who comes into our office full of doubts and misgivings. He thinks that he might want to be at the birth, but then again he thinks he might not. How might his question be answered?

Father: Doctor, Molly and I are going to these classes, and we've talked about, you know, that I might be there in the delivery room, and it's not like anything I've heard about before from other people. How do you feel about it? What do you think?

Physician: Well, no one should be forced into the delivery room, and I can understand that you might have reservations. What is it exactly that makes you think that you shouldn't be there?

Father: Well, I don't know. I just had this feeling that you might not want me there. I thought I might just be in the way or that the doctors had their thing to do, they had their job to do, and I just maybe didn't belong there. I just wouldn't fit in with what you have to do.

Physician: Do you feel that you would be unable to help your wife during the labor and birth?

Father: Well, I don't know, doctor. I don't really know what to do. I don't want to be in the way.

Physician: There are a lot of men who feel that they'll just be in the way, and that's not true. We will teach you all about what's going on and what you can be doing to help your wife.

"Why am I needed"

Father: But why am I needed there, anyway? I mean, my wife's here having the baby and I'm not, so why should I be in there, anyway?

Physician: Today we feel that if the father isn't there, something's missing. It's almost like there's a vacuum created—something isn't there that ought to be. We have come to realize that a woman does much better in labor and birth if the father is with her. She is less frightened, less alone. He is the one person who is unalterably on her side, the person to whom she can talk and express her feelings and who is not there, potentially, to hurt her.

We have found that fathers are a tremendous help. With a few words they can support their wives who are nervous and tense or getting a little bit out of control. Just a few words like "Relax, you're breathing too fast," can be all it takes. They give the woman both physical and emotional support, and this makes it easier for the doctor, too. In the past, women had to depend on the hospital staff for emotional support. A lot of times it wasn't easy or possible for the staff to get involved to that point, to really give women all the emotional support they needed. They needed a real coach because it takes a certain amount of training, and you have to be involved with that person to transfer emotional support. We will give you that training so that you can coach your wife and help her in this way.

I think when you get to the hospital you'll find an excellent nursing staff, all trained in prepared childbirth techniques. If for any reason during the labor you wish to leave, or if you feel that you need some help in coaching your wife, these trained people may take over for you or give you the encouragement you need to help your wife. They will give you any help that you need.

There are no regulations; there's nothing to keep you there, and no one restricts your movement. There will be some tables that are sterile that you can't touch without wearing sterile gloves and gowns, but other than that, you're not restricted in the room.

We feel that you're an important part of this whole thing. If you're down the hall in a room somewhere, there's no way for you to participate in this exciting event, which most people only have one or two chances in their whole lifetime to experience.

"But I'll be nervous!"

Father: I'll be so nervous!

Physician: Once they are in the labor and delivery room, most men fit in very quickly. Even nervous individuals usually do extremely well. And then, like I said, there are a lot of people who will support you.

Father: Is my wife going to be nervous?

Physician: I don't think so. Your wife is going to be concentrating a great deal on the job that she has to do. That's where you really can help because you can help her concentrate.

"Will I be able to talk?"

Father: Will I be able to talk when I'm there, or do I just have to keep still?

Physician: You can talk all you want to. There isn't anyone whom you're going to bother in the delivery room.

"Won't it be bloody?"

Father: You know, I just remembered talking to my dad one time, and he said he was sure glad he didn't have to go in there and see all that bloody mess and all that. They'd never get him in there. I was thinking, don't men feel that way, other men?

Physician: In the classes you will have seen films of at least two births that are very typical of what your wife's childbirth will be like. Sometimes the birth is very slow and difficult, but usually it's really fast and exciting. There might be a lot of blood, but it shouldn't bother you at all. After all, your wife during the process of nine months of pregnancy has made about two extra pints of blood, and so you expect her to lose it. Nature expects her to lose some blood at that time. Really, everything has been geared up and prepared for that, so she's just losing what nature expects her to lose. The important thing is that the classes will prepare you to understand everything that's going on. When you understand it, and know *why* it happens, then it won't bother you at all.

"What if something goes wrong?"

Father: What if something goes wrong in there?

Physician: Well, a complication is really quite rare, but I'm sure you understand that if there is a problem, I'll do my best to take care of it. If you're asked to leave the delivery room, I'm sure you will. But most of the time, you won't be asked to leave the room unless there is a cesarean section or something like that because I think you ought to be able to appreciate whatever goes on. With the things you will learn in the classes, you'll be prepared to understand just about everything that might happen there.

Father: Don't you think I might get angry with you if something happens?

Physician: No, not at all.

Father: Why not? I mean, I might blame you or something.

Physician: Well, as long as you can see that I am doing my best to help your wife and your baby, I just can't imagine your being angry. Incidentally, everything that is done will be explained. For example, if an IV is started, I might tell you that medication must be given because the uterus is soft and it has to contract so your wife will stop bleeding. I will explain things so that you will understand and not have to ask why something is being done.

Since you bring up this matter of something going wrong, and you seem to be worried about my feelings in having you there if that happens, I'm going to tell you something from my own experience. Of course, this is something very rare, but it serves to illustrate a point.

I was caring for a woman once who had a very normal labor. She had no anesthesia, no episiotomy, her labor and delivery went very smoothly without any interference. When the baby was born, he had a normal heart rate but he just didn't start breathing. No matter how much work and effort was put forth, the baby wouldn't breathe.

The pediatrician and I spent half an hour trying to resuscitate the baby. During this whole time the woman was certainly wide awake and her husband was there with her in the delivery room. When it got to the point where it was simply impossible to do anything more for the child, both of the parents actually thanked me and consoled me. They thanked me for all the effort that we put forth trying to save their baby. Can you imagine? It was their baby who had died, but *they* were consoling me!

As I left the delivery room and started down the hall, I thought what a tremendously different experience it would have been in the past. I would now have to go to the Father's Room and tell the father that his baby died, and then try to explain to him why. His wife would have been still under anesthesia at that point, and she would not yet have known about the death of her child. I might never have been able to make those parents really understand how hard we had tried. As I thought back to the way it used to be, I was very glad that *this* time both the parents were wide awake and right there watching. It was really so much easier for me—and easier for them too.

"What about after the baby is born?"

Father: OK, let's say I'm going to be there and I'm going to be helping with the birth. What about after the baby is born? What happens then?

Physician: After the baby is born, he is wiped dry and then handed to your wife. That's quite an experience for her—to be able to touch the baby. The baby will be warm, really warm, with a kind of unusual odor that you won't forget. As soon as the baby is wrapped up and warm, with the mother holding him, he will stop crying.

Father: I could hold the baby right then! And then you would take him away and put him in one of those baskets in the room, is that right?

Physician: Not if you want to hold him. If you wish to continue holding the baby for a while you can if the baby's temperature remains normal. He doesn't have to go into the isolette at all.

Father: Does the baby have to be taken to the nursery?

Physician: Not unless you want the baby to go to the nursery.

Father: You mean he can be with my wife and me the whole time?

Physician: From the time he's born until he leaves the hospital.

Father: I've been in those hospitals and seen all those baskets lined up, and I just thought that's how it was.

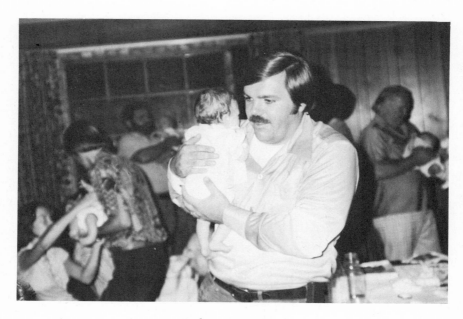

Enthusiasm started.

Physician: Things have changed a lot in the last few years. But even now, people vary a lot in what they want to do. Some people wish to experience the whole occasion, while others don't want to remember anything from the time they get to the hospital until the next day. There are some individuals who want to have their babies with them all the time, and others who want them brought out just for feedings. You can't set up one policy and expect everybody to fit into that mold. What we do is to set up criteria and guidelines and then let people select what they want. It's up to you to decide what you wish to do. Everybody, including the doctor, is much happier that way.

Some individuals leave the hospital within 2 or 3 hours after the baby is born. I don't think that's a good policy because it really takes about 24 hours for the baby to get stabilized and to see that he's not going to have any problems. That's a good reason in itself for the woman to stay in the hospital for a day, but there's no reason why the baby can't stay with you and your wife during that whole period of time. A pediatrician will come and examine the baby, and the nurses periodically will come in and see that the baby is doing well.

You see, it's really up to you, but my own feeling is that this experience is one of the most important moments in your life, and that it belongs to you.

UNIT III

Family-centered care

THE FAMILY

> Only the mother-to-be is admitted to a maternity unit, but the nurse is admitting to care not one but three persons—mother, father, and infant— each dependent on the other for a safe and memorable birth. At no time during the childbearing experience should any person in this three-sided unit be lost sight of, for exclusion of one member of the family can have serious consequences for all.*

The childbearing family begins labor emotionally welded together, sharing the common goal of a safe and memorable birth experience. Each family member has needs and expectations, realistic or not, and the action of each individual family member has an effect on the entire family.

In the nineteenth century and in the early part of the twentieth century, it was common to find several generations living together in joint families, which could include all living descendants. In such an "extended family" the childbearing couple received much support from family members. Although the new mother did not have an automatic washer and dryer to keep the baby's diapers clean, she had her grandmother or a great aunt or sister to help with the chores. And, of course, the new father had many family members to help him in his new

---

*From Phillips, C.: The essence of birth without violence, MCN The American Journal of Maternal Child Nursing, pp. 162–163, May/June, 1976.

37

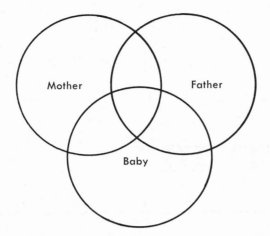

The family triad.

role. The information shared had been tested and improved, and "home remedies" had been validated for generations. There was a closeness and a feeling of belonging in these families, softening the adjustment to parenthood.

However, particularly since World War II, family life in United States culture has changed to small nuclear units, consisting of the mother, father, and children who often live many miles away from other family members. Technology may have given modern parents mechanical servants to keep the diapers clean; however, these mechanical marvels give no emotional support and share little information on infant care.

In reaction to the rapidly changing world of today, some couples are returning to the extended family by developing communities of their own, sometimes termed *communes*, which have all the dimensions of a family. Childbearing couples in such a community have support systems that the couple in a nuclear family seldom has.

The more nuclear a family becomes, and the fewer support systems they have, the more important it is to meet the needs of each family member during the birth process. This could be a critical time for them to build their concepts of themselves as a family.[10]

TRADITIONAL MATERNITY CARE

Since maternity care in the United States traditionally has been centered in hospitals that are dedicated to treating sickness and curing disease, it has often suffered under the rigid organizational structure of the pathology-oriented institution. Although 85% to 90% of pregnancies are perfectly normal, the childbearing woman is often subjected to hospital routines identical to those for someone who is ill while she is being admitted to a traditional hospital room to labor. When she is ready to give birth, this woman is transferred to a delivery room, which could also function as a major surgery room. The environment of a hospital birth in the United States for many couples is cold, sterile, often lonely, but worst of all, depersonalized.

Perhaps the best way to understand what it may be like to experience birth in a traditional hospital setting today would be to imagine how you might feel in a typical situation.

Imagine yourself standing in front of a hospital admissions desk, holding a small suitcase with your possessions in it. You feel excited, even though you are tired. Labor began 5 hours ago with uterine cramping and a backache.

The cramps became harder as the hours passed, until now your uterus is contracting hard every 3 to 4 minutes, and the feeling of tightness and pressure lasts a full minute each time as your backache increases in intensity.

The father of your baby is signing hospital admission forms and answering questions about plans to pay the bill. You listen only because you feel that talking would take too much energy now, and besides, you are trying to concentrate on relaxing with each contraction, as you have practiced for months.

A nurse's aide arrives with a wheelchair and asks you to sit in it so she may take you to the Labor Unit. You feel silly being pushed down the corridor in a wheelchair. After all, don't they know you are not sick, or an invalid, or anything? The thought of how silly this parade must look almost makes you laugh as you turn around to see the expectant father walking on behind, juggling admission forms and your suitcase.

One more uterine contraction comes while you are on your way to the Labor Unit, and you wish you could relax better.

The Labor Unit is entered through double doors marked DELIVERY ROOMS—NO ADMITTANCE, and a nurse greets you, helping you out of the wheelchair, while asking yet a third person in a plain-looking cotton dress to "admit you." It seems busy in the corridor; several men in white cotton suits are walking in and out of small rooms, frowning, and various uniformed people are moving equipment across the corridor.

You are alone now. Your partner who has practiced breathing exercises with you has been sent to wait in a Father's Waiting Room, outside the unit, while you are admitted. The contractions seem to be every few minutes now, and they are intense. While you try to relax, this

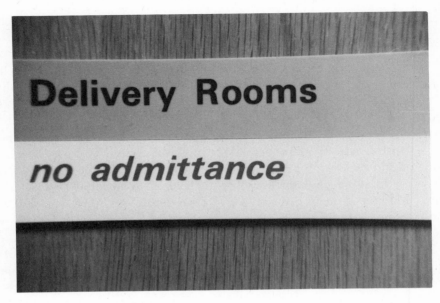

No admittance.

new nurse has placed a thermometer in your mouth, making it very difficult to breathe out through pursed lips, as you had practiced. Things are happening fast. You have taken off all your clothing and stand naked, a bit chilled, waiting for a small gown that ties in the back, leaving your entire backside exposed. How undignified! And how ugly you feel! You have always enjoyed colorful, soft nightgowns, and this coarse, gray thing is indescribable. It matches the plain white-gray room and narrow hospital bed with those strange cranks at the bottom that look to you like some torture device from the late, late movie. At last the thermometer is gone so that you can breathe again. Oh, the pressure! It feels like a ton of bricks on your abdomen, making it difficult to breathe.

There are more questions about what you have brought with you and lists of possessions to sign. What does it matter? They have taken everything away. You feel so alone. Now the nurse explains that she will shave you and give you an enema. What an embarrassing moment! You look at the ceiling, praying she has a sharp razor, trying to ignore the position you are in and hoping no one walks in now. This nurse must be experienced because before another contraction is over, she tells you to turn on your side for the enema. This is a new experience. As the water fills your lower bowel, you feel like you will surely burst. There can't be any room left down there! But the nurse finds an inch. Ooh! And now to the bathroom. . . . Your uterus contracts again at the same time that you have to expel the enema water. It hurts. Everything hurts. The childbirth teacher didn't say it would be like this. Where is your coach? Why can't he be here to help? It's so hard to stay relaxed, now. Here comes another nurse, just to look in on you—"On the toilet yet?"

At last, it's over. You can go back and climb up into that high, narrow bed. The nurse is waiting to examine you vaginally. Wow! The antiseptic solution she pours over your bottom is so cold, and her fingers are so long. Where did she come from anyway? She must be the third or fourth person whom you have met since entering this hospital. How many are there? Aren't hospitals understaffed, like all the newspapers report? These nurses all look alike—in those outfits they call "scrub dresses."

Where is your coach? There he is, a worried look on his pale face. He has been given permission to join you now that you are officially admitted. Strange as it may seem, you feel grateful and thank everyone. You need him so, and maybe if you are supersweet, they will let him stay.

Time has no meaning now—just the contractions, one after another. It's hot. The walls seem to close in, as though the room were a tunnel.

In the next room a girl cries out loudly, "Help me, help me!" You wish that she'd be quiet. What's wrong with her? Is she dying? Didn't Great-grandmother die in childbirth? Maybe you will too.

The shift has changed, and there are all new nurses now. How many of these new ones are there?

Where is the doctor? He only came in to see you during lunchtime, and that must have been days ago. No, not really. It has only been 5 hours that you have been here, but when you are working as hard as you are, it seems like days.

You are working as a team with your partner now, relaxing, using fast chest breathing. If only you could get up and walk around or even get up on all fours, maybe that would help the backache. But hospital policy says you may not walk around because your membranes are ruptured, and the bed is so high that you may fall if you get up on all fours.

Occasionally, nurses bring nursing students in to watch your team-work with comments on how well you are doing. Why don't they leave you alone? It is so hard to concentrate and be polite, too.

You are so tired now and so thirsty. But you may not have a drink—hospital policy, just in case you need an anesthetic. You wouldn't want to choke on vomit, they say. Ugh! Now you really feel nauseated.

There is a strange new feeling beginning—an urge to push. It's unbearable. You must push! And when you do, the strange sounds you make are scary, gutteral, loud—almost like an animal. They have closed the door to the room because of the noise, and now the hot, stale air in the small room is choking.

This narrow, white room with its shiny walls and antiseptic smell is closing in on you. Nurses and students and doctors are coming and going, waiting to see "50 cents worth of head." Why don't they do something? This is their place, they know all, and you are so tired.

Your partner looks helpless now, searching the face of each new person who walks into the room. It's as though he wants an answer, too. They know what to do. Why don't they do it? You really wouldn't care now. You are theirs.

At last it's time to be moved to the delivery room, across the corridor, past more faces. Who are they? Now lift up and over, onto the delivery table. Not now! Please wait until this contraction is over.

Push, push! Where is he! Why isn't he here? He can't come in because there may be a problem with the baby? What? Why? Who are all the people in the room? Students? Pediatrician? Nurses?

Push, push! Oh, you feel like your bottom will split . . . red hot! Look, see the baby's head is born. Is he all right? Why doesn't he cry? What are they doing to him? Why doesn't someone answer?

Oh, thank God, he cried. He's going to be all right, but they'll have to take him to the nursery now. You can see him tomorrow. Don't worry, mother. Mother? Me a mother? I feel so tired, just let me rest.

By now, you are probably feeling impatient, perhaps resenting the little scenario, thinking it was overdramatized and even sensationalized. Perhaps it was, and then, perhaps it wasn't. It all depends on where the birth occurred because policies, procedure, and attitudes regarding birth differ drastically in hospitals throughout the United States.

If you are a medical person, dealing daily with birth, you may be feeling angry now because as the story ended, you became aware of the sense of urgency—of emergency. And then you realized that the story had a happy ending and that the happy ending was because of all the skills that were used. What had been a normal labor for an apparently normal mother became an emergency, threatening the life and degree of wellness of the unborn child as the cord, wrapped around the baby's neck three times, tightened when the mother pushed. An alert nurse, listening to fetal heart tones almost constantly, detected immediately the decelerating, falling heart rate. Responding quickly, she alerted the rest of the maternity team, and the drama unfolded. It was necessary for a skilled physician to enlarge the vaginal opening with an incision, then apply forceps to the baby's head, assisting the final rotation so that the baby could be born quickly. Even before the head emerged the physician had partially freed the tight cord, clamped and cut it, so that the baby emerged free of the strangling noose. The team of pediatricians, responding to an emergency call, stood by and skillfully and gently resuscitated the depressed baby.

Yes, those medical teams deserve congratulations. All of their years of training, their diverse knowledge, and their skills came into play as they worked wordlessly side by side. This was the "insurance" that the couple had purchased when paying for the high-priced maternity care of today. And their policy had paid off.

But what of their feelings? How are they feeling about being parents? What has this birth meant to them? This is the beginning of a family for them. The mother is "alone" in the delivery room, confused, frightened, and still wondering what happened. The father is "alone" in the waiting room, apprehensive, puzzled, and angry at being rushed out of the way. And the baby is in an intensive care nursery, dazed, looking at the plastic wall of an isolette, listening to the whirr of the motor, also "alone."

WHAT A PRICE TO PAY FOR SUCCESS!

Traditional maternity care in the United States is compartmentalized, fragmented, bound in routines, depersonalized, and occurs within the context of major surgery. A laboring woman is admitted to a labor and delivery unit, with one set of personnel, transferred to a recovery room, sometimes staffed with its own personnel, and then transferred to a postpartum unit, with yet another staff. Unless there are rooming-in provisions, the baby is transferred to a nursery, staffed by entirely different personnel.[15] Not only does the mother have to relate to numerous people but she has to relate to numerous messages from them. Because of the compartmentalization of the maternity service, the nurses have become specialists within their units, and they find it safe to maintain this specialty. The mother is passed from hand to hand and literally caught betwixt and between. If her questions do not fall within its area of expertise, one department refers her to the next for answers. If the hospital has a rooming-in policy, the father is not considered to be a visitor and may come and go as he wishes. He may be present as his baby feeds and may hold and interact with his child, thus beginning the bonding process.[5] However, even in these units hospital routines often dictate that demonstrations of infant care are given in the morning or afternoon while the father is at work and cannot be present.

If the hospital does not have a rooming-in policy, the father is restricted to visiting with his family during visiting hours, which may be in direct conflict with his working hours. In such regimentation he may not touch his baby or even be present during feeding time. This father's hospital contact with his own baby is made through the glass "observing" windows of a nursery.

It is important that the other children be given the opportunity to visit their mother while she is in the hospital. This will be comforting not only to the mother but also to the young siblings and help to minimize their feelings of abandonment. In addition, sibling visitation will foster early bonding with the new brother or sister.

As hospital costs rise, the length of hospital stay for maternity care goes down. It simply becomes a matter of economic necessity for women to go home as soon as they are able. Unfortunately, the new family usually goes home from the institution just described barely prepared for parenting and uninformed about how to deal with the normal physiological changes that the new mother will experience in the first postpartum days. Without having members of an extended family to help, many young couples are left to their own resources until the first postpartum checkup with the physician at four to six weeks after the birth.[11]

As childbearing couples are becoming better informed, childbirth is becoming demystified and recognized for the normal process that it is 85% to 90% of the time.[7] Movements to humanize the way of birth in the United States are growing, and there is considerable evidence that this desire for making each birth unique, occurring in an atmosphere of joy and dignity, will not be a passing trend.[13] Birth at home is an option that some couples are choosing as a way out of a situation they find intolerable.[6] The California Bureau of Maternal and Child Health continues to receive more and more requests for information on home birth services.[13]

In an era of rapidly expanding technology and an explosion of knowledge, society has come too far to deny unborn generations the benefits of this advanced body of knowledge. Modern medicine and modern medical education have the tools and skills to make birth both safe and humane. A return to home birth without skilled supervision and, most important, without skilled backup involves unnecessary risks to mother and infant.[2]

The answer is not to boycott the present system but to change it to provide relevant maternity care. It is possible to have the best of both worlds—modern perinatology and humanistic, homelike care at the same time by developing safe and acceptable options in maternity care within the hospital setting.

MATERNITY CARE ALTERNATIVES

The planning of maternity care alternatives should begin by a close inspection and evaluation of the maternity delivery system presently in operation. The involvement of prospective parents and new parents in this initial process is vital. Maternity care should no longer be based on stereotyped or ritualistic procedures.

It is true that "Maternal and child health nursing practice is characterized by the continual questioning of the assumptions upon which practice is based, retaining those which are valid and searching for and using new knowledge."*

After this initial examination and evaluation of each hospital maternity policy and procedure, those which are not based on scientific fact as required by law should be considered for revision objectively, systematically, and logically.

It is essential to keep in mind all childbearing families when planning care and to keep safe care always the top priority.

Those families who require top-level medical intervention should have all the sophisticated medical tools, facilities, and support systems needed, which may mean standard hospital rooms and standard delivery rooms and operating rooms. Whereas those families who do not have serious medical problems should be able to choose a homelike atmosphere in which to labor, give birth, and recover, and it should take place in close proximity to support systems for handling any emergency.

There are pioneering "models of care" in operation now both on the East and West Coasts and in the middle of the United States.[4,8,14] Since maternity care professionals are caught in the middle of "future shock," to name each courageous pioneer would be to risk obsolescence before publication. As the utilization of these centers grows, it will become increasingly clear that birth can be safe for all families and still occur in an atmosphere of joy and dignity.

Alternative Birth Centers

In contrast to the birth just described, birth within one of the new Alternative Birth Centers was described as follows in the *San Francisco Chronicle.*[6]

Sarah Katherine Bell was born at 8:56 P.M. Tuesday, May 11, at Mount Zion Hospital. Unlike the experience of her 4 year old brother,

*From Standards of maternal-child nursing practice, The American Nurse, p. 16, July, 1974.

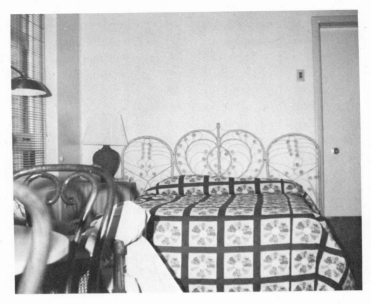

Birth bed in Alternative Birth Center.
(Courtesy Mount Zion Hospital, San Francisco.)

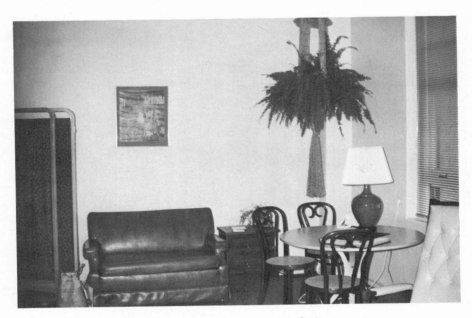

One corner of Alternative Birth Center.
(Courtesy Mount Zion Hospital, San Francisco.)

Sarah's first glimpse of the world was not a sterile delivery room bathed in harsh light and filled with the latest medical equipment, but a room that could have been anyone's bedroom.

Her mother, Judy, delivered in a standard double bed with a wicker headboard. Around the bed were plants suspended from macrame hangers, an orange carpet and a sofabed where her father, Tami, could relax when he wasn't coaching his wife's breathing. The lights were low and there was a stereo system for music.

Soon after Sarah's birth, Tami picked up the couple's son from a babysitter and brought him to the hospital to meet and touch his new sister. By the next morning the Bells were ready to take their baby home.°

Sarah Bell was the first baby born in the new Alternative Birth Center at Mount Zion Hospital in San Francisco. This center was developed to provide the intimate, relaxed atmosphere of a home birth in the hospital setting, accompanied by the staff and equipment to care for any unexpected complications.[3]

The setting of the Alternative Birth Center is homelike, consisting of a

°From Home birth at the hospital, *San Francisco Chronicle,* June 8, 1976; copyright Chronicle Publishing Co.

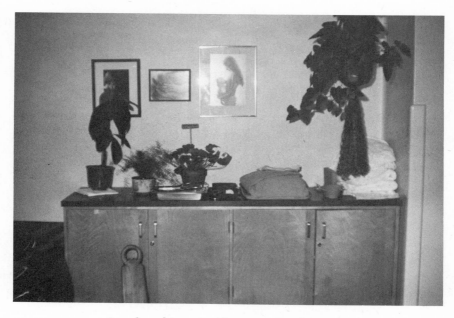

Supply cabinets in Alternative Birth Center.
(Courtesy Mount Zion Hospital, San Francisco.)

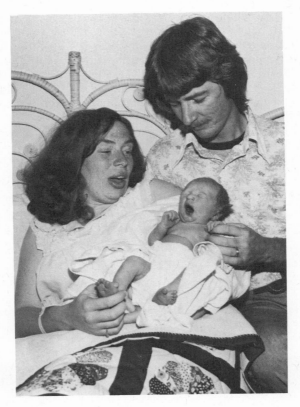

A new family.
(Courtesy Mount Zion Hospital, San Francisco.)

room or maternity unit that has been cheerfully and comfortably furnished. The family is admitted to this room, labors there, gives birth there, and may remain there until discharge if the time interval and requirements for room utilization permit. If the family has to remain in the hospital for more than 24 hours postpartum, the demand for use of the Alternative Birth Center by more prospective families may require transfer of the new family to a regular postpartum room.

Ideally, the Alternative Birth Center becomes the private space for one childbearing family throughout their birth experience and until they are ready to go home. It is a warm, private, friendly space within a complex, fully equipped medical constellation. All medicines and equipment that may be needed for normal obstetrical care are stored out of sight in cabinets and cupboards that are tastefully incorporated into the decor of the room. When birth is imminent, the necessary equipment

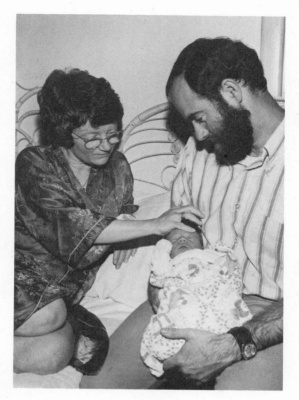

Private space for a childbearing family.
(Courtesy Mount Zion Hospital, San Francisco.)

and supplies can be brought out of their storage places and be put to use as needed. The mother gives birth, positioning herself to meet her comfort needs, on the large, low double bed. Beanbag chairs, stools, pillows, towels, and foam bolsters are all available to her to help support her back and make her comfortable.

A nurse from the Alternative Birth Center staff comes into the hospital and stays with the family throughout the labor and birth and for several hours after the birth. Since all of the center's nurses are present at orientation sessions attended by the families before birth, the nurse has already met the couple before D Day. Within 24 hours after birth two home visits to the family are made by the same nurse to check the baby and provide support to the family. Thus continuity of care is provided, and the family does not have to relate to large numbers of nurses and hospital personnel at a time when they are in need of consistent support systems.

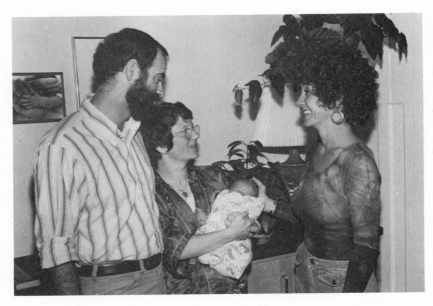

Alternative Birth Center family with their nurse.
(Courtesy Mount Zion Hospital, San Francisco.)

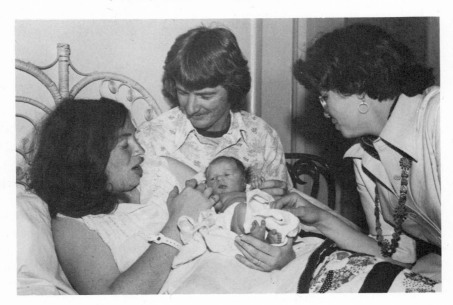

Together.
(Courtesy Mount Zion Hospital, San Francisco.)

Throughout their stay in the Alternative Birth Center the mother and baby are not separated unless absolutely necessary. If the couple wishes to have their other child or children with them during this experience, this is possible, too. However, there must be provision for care of this child or children at all times and their preparation for the birth experience must be assured. Alternative Birth Centers often permit other family members and friends to visit.

Alternative Birth Centers are beginning to meet the needs of a growing number of consumers who have expressed dissatisfaction with traditional hospital maternity care. The people who choose to give birth in such a center must play an active role in assuming responsibility for their labor, birth, and postpartum care. The mother-to-be must be classified as a "normal" patient, must be receiving prenatal care, and must be participating in childbirth classes. In addition to childbirth classes the childbearing family must attend orientation sessions conducted by the staff of the Alternative Birth Center to become familiar with the facilities and procedures. At these orientation sessions the center staff can also get to know the family and learn of their expectations. The emphasis is on normalcy, family involvement, and participation in decision making in a nontraditional environment that can be personalized.

While emphasizing normalcy, natural methods, self-help, and family participation, Alternative Birth Centers are fully supported by the presence of an obstetrical nurse or nurse-midwife and by the availability of obstetrical and pediatric house staff at all times, with attending staff backup.

If a situation that could threaten the safety of the mother or baby should arise at any time in labor, the mother would be moved to the regular labor and delivery area. In such a situation the Alternative Birth Center nurse and the father of the baby would also go with her.

Families who choose birth in the Alternative Birth Center may experience a warm, positive, family-centered, highly personalized, highly emotional birth within a structure offering safe and preventitive perinatal care. Immediately outside the door of their "alternative birth space," this family has available to them the sophistication of technical resources for management of complicated obstetrical situations—truly the best of two worlds!

An Alternative Birth Center does not just happen; it is the result of extensive planning and retraining of all personnel involved. Studies and surveys of the local community must be done to determine the specific needs of the childbearing population, as well as the resources available to develop a viable alternative to traditional labor and birth.

Ideally, an Alternative Birth Center should also offer childbearing couples alternative prices, in contrast to the high cost of obstetrical care. Since alternative birth requires that the family occupy fewer spaces, less hospital time, and fewer supplies, linen, staff, and so on, it is usually possible to reduce the overall cost of birth to hospital and consumer.

The establishment of an Alternative Birth Center requires the hospital maternity personnel, childbirth educators, physicians, and parents to come together to develop a common philosophy out of which can be elicited specific goals and objectives. The next step is to develop specific policies and procedures to provide uniform standards that will achieve the designated goals. An example of criteria relative to a couple's admission to an Alternative Birth Center follows.*

High-risk factors excluding admission to the Alternative Birth Center

Social factors
  Three prenatal visits
  Maternal age: primipara, 35 years of age; multipara, 40 years of age
Preexisting maternal disease
  Chronic hypertension
  Moderate or severe renal disease
  Heart disease, Classes II to IV
  History of toxemia with seizures
  Diabetes
  Anemia; + hemoglobin 9.5 gm/100 ml†
  Tuberculosis
  Chronic or acute pulmonary problem
  Psychiatric disease requiring major tranquilizer
Previous obstetrical history
  Previous stillbirth
  Previous cesarean section
  Rh sensitization
  Multiparity 5†
  Previous infant with respiratory distress syndrome at same gestation
Present pregnancy
  Toxemia
  Gestational age of 37 or 42 weeks
  Multiple pregnancy
  Abnormal presentation (primipara with floating head will need evaluation
    by obstetrician)
  Third trimester bleeding or known placenta previa

---

*From Alternative Birth Center policies and procedures, San Francisco, Calif., April, 1976, Mount Zion Hospital and Medical Center, Department of Obstetrics and Pediatrics.
†May use center with IV during labor.

Prolonged ruptured membranes, 24 hours

Estimated fetal weight of < 5 or > 9 pounds

Contracted pelvis, any plane

Pelvic pathology, e.g., adnexal masses, uterine malformation, polyhydramnios, pelvic tumors, genital herpes

Treatment with reserpine, lithium, or magnesium

Induction

Spinal or epidural anesthesia

Any other acute or chronic maternal illness, which in opinion of medical
staff would increase risk to mother or infant

**High-risk factors developing after admission requiring transfer to labor
and delivery***

Hemoglobin: 9.5 gm/100 ml†

Temperature 38° C

Significant variation of maternal blood pressure from previously recorded
values in office; fall or rise of maternal blood pressure of greater than 30/15
mm Hg

Deeply stained meconium in amniotic fluid

Abnormal fetal heart rate or pattern

Prolonged true labor for 24 hours

Arrest of labor in active phase

Second stage labor for 2 hours for primipara, 1 hour for multipara

Significant vaginal bleeding

Development of any factor that requires continuous fetal heart rate monitoring

Any labor pattern or maternal or fetal complication that attending physician or
nurse believes requires more sophisticated diagnosis or treatment than can
be done in Alternative Birth Center.

Just as well-defined criteria for admission must be developed,
guidelines for participation of family members must be designed. An
example of such guidelines follows.

Guidelines for participation of siblings and others

1. All children must be prepared to share this experience.
2. All children under 12 years of age must be accompanied by an adult who is
   not considered a major support person and who can leave with the children
   if this becomes necessary (mother becomes high risk, child very upset,
   child ill).
3. All children must be screened, including temperature for current infectious
   process. A gown must be worn after scrubbing if the baby is to be
   touched.
4. Children must be entertained in the center (not allowed in halls).
5. Food and toys for children should be brought from home.

---

*Should a problem resolve, the woman may be transferred back to the Alternative Birth
Center or give birth in the labor room.
†Must have IV during labor.

6. Consideration of the newborn must be observed; that is, an ill or difficult-to-manage child may not come to the center.
7. The specific plan for family participation must have been approved by the center staff prior to admission to the center.

Other participants

1. Consideration for the comfort and safety of mother and infant must be the first priority.
2. The number of others should have prior approval, and it should be understood that they may be asked to leave if their presence seems to be stressful to the laboring mother and support person assisting her (father, other major helper) or if the mother must be moved out of the center.
3. All others and visitors will be screened simply by the nurse in attendance.
4. Anyone who will come in contact with the newborn must scrub for 3 minutes and then gown prior to the birth.

Criteria for immediate rooming-in and for early discharge of both mother and baby follow.

Criteria for immediate rooming-in (mother and infant will remain in center together)

Initial evaluation of infant
Five-minute Apgar score of 7 or over
Weight over 5 or under 9.5 pounds
Vital signs normal (heart rate 110 to 170 beats/min; respirations 35 to 70 breaths/min)
Color normal
Airway open, including nares
Suction catheter passes to stomach
Vitamin K given
Silver nitrate administered to eyes
Complete papers
Observation period (4 to 6 hours)
Frequent observations during first hour
Vital signs qh × 4, then q4h
Hematocrit and Dextrostix at 4 hours
Blood type, Coombs test, and Rh test if mother is Rh negative or blood type O
Nurse present for first feeding
Visitors at discretion of hospital personnel, depending on time of day, ward schedule, space available, and number of people

Criteria for early discharge

Infant (between 10 A.M. and 10 P.M.)
Not less than 6 hours post partum; birth weight over 5 or under 9.5 pounds
Vital signs stable; temperature 36.50 to 37.50 C; heart rate 110 to 160 beats/min; respirations 30 to 60 breaths/min

Physical examination normal; to be done by pediatric house officer or private pediatrician

Hematocrit 45% to 65%; Dextrostix 45 mg/100 ml or more

Blood type and Coombs test show no evidence of incompatibility

No complication requiring additional observation

At least one water feeding and/or two formula or breast feedings

Mother must demonstrate ability to handle and care for infant

Birth certificate complete

Home care record understood

Home care record

Parents maintain notes of the following:

Infant's first voiding if not in hospital; notify if not by 24 hours

First meconium stool; if not by 36 hours, notify pediatrician

Feedings

Any changes in infant

A home visit should be made by the nurse in the first 24 hours and on day 3. On the day 3 visit the nurse will draw PKU and bilirubin if indicated, or the mother may take the infant to the pediatric clinic or private pediatrician.

Mother

No medical complications requiring close supervision (e.g., cardiovascular problems, diabetes, etc.)

No antepartum or intrapartum obstetrical complications requiring close postpartum observation (e.g., toxemia, hemorrhage, signs of infection, etc.)

Length of labor: less than 30 hours for primipara; less than 24 hours for multipara

Ruptured membranes less than 24 hours

Perineum: episiotomy or less than third-degree lacerations, no hematoma formation, or unusually severe bruising

Blood loss less than 500 ml

Delivery spontaneous or low forceps

Analgesia/anesthesia: mother with spinal, caudal, epidural, or general anesthesia not to be discharged in less than 24 hours

Postpartum course

Vital signs: temperature less than 38° C; pulse less than 100 beats/min; blood pressure more than 90/60 mm Hg, less than 140/90 mm Hg, and consistent with prenatal course

Fundus firm with no excessive bleeding

Hematocrit more than 32% or hemoglobin more than 10.5 gm/100 ml

Able to ambulate easily and care for self and baby

Able to void adequately

Rho-GAM eligibility determined and plan for administration developed

Plan for assistance at home for at least 2 days

As Alternative Birth Centers are developing in progressive hospitals throughout the United States, various other alternatives to traditional hospital maternity care are also proliferating. There is a steady increase in home births, attended by midwives and physicians or simply by the family itself.[8] In many hospitals nurse-midwifery services are successful and growing.[7] Demonstration projects are being developed to offer out-of-hospital maternity care in a homelike setting for the low-risk, childbearing population. In these models the care is provided by an obstetrician/nurse-midwife team.[7]

Since excellent books have been written on these alternatives to traditional care and since we believe that safe alternative care should be offered within the hospital setting, they will be mentioned only briefly here.

As these new and well-planned programs for the "normal" childbearing population increase, we believe that maternity care providers will respond to improve the experience of the family while continuing to offer the family the best standards of safety available. We feel certain that the establishment of Alternative Birth Centers is the beginning of this response—the beginning of the maternity health care system's new consciousness.

However, as with all change, the transition process will be slow and difficult, and will meet with much resistance. As maternity services become more relevant to the needs, ideas, and interests of the family, the father will play a more active part, fulfilling his natural role as parent. When this happens, family-centered care will take on its true meaning, responding to the needs of all members of an expectant family.

REFERENCES

1. Alternative Birth Center policies and procedures, San Francisco, Calif., April, 1976, Mount Zion Hospital and Medical Center, Department of Obstetrics and Pediatrics.
2. American College of Obstetricians and Gynecologists District II.: Position paper on out-of-hospital maternity care, ICEA News **15:**2-3, Spring, 1976.
3. An Alternative Birth Center, San Francisco, Calif., April, 1976, Mount Zion Hospital and Medical Center.
4. Bear, M.: Birth is a family affair, American Journal of Nursing **75:**1689, 1975.
5. Haire, D., and Haire, J.: Implementing family-centered maternity care with a central nursery, Hillside, N.J., 1971, International Childbirth Education Association, Inc.
6. Home birth at the hospital, San Francisco Chronicle, June 8, 1976.
7. Lubic, R.: Developing maternity services women will trust, American Journal of Nursing **75:**1686, 1975.
8. Maternity care alternatives. New Life Center and Booth Maternity Center, ICEA News **14:**1-5, Winter, 1975.
9. Phillips, C.: The essence of birth without violence, MCN The American Journal of Maternal Child Nursing, pp. 162-163, May/June, 1976.
10. Rising, S. S.: The fourth stage of labor: family integration, American Journal of Nursing **74:**870-874, 1974..
11. Rubin, R.: Maternity nursing stops too soon, American Journal of Nursing **75:**1684, 1975.
12. Standards of maternal-child nursing practice, The American Nurse, p. 16, July, 1974.

13. The health professional role in relation to home birth, Family Health Bulletin **14:**1-5, Summer, 1971.

14. Timberlake, B.: The New Life Center, American Journal of Nursing **75:**1457, 1975.

15. Walker, L.: Providing more relevant maternity services, Journal of Obstetric, Gynecologic and Neonatal Nursing, p. 34, March/April, 1974.

ADDITIONAL READINGS

Arms, S.: Immaculate deception: a new look at women and childbirth, Boston, 1975, Houghton Mifflin Co.

Bean, C. A.: Methods of childbirth, Garden City, N.Y., 1972, Doubleday and Co.

Boston Women's Health Book Collective, Inc.: Our bodies, ourselves, New York, 1973, Simon and Schuster.

Hazell, L. D.: Common sense childbirth, New York, 1969, G. P. Putnam's Sons.

Shaw, N. S.: Forced labor: maternity care in the United States, Elmsford, N.Y., 1974, Pergamon Press.

Sousa, M.: Childbirth at home, Englewood Cliffs, N.J., 1976, Prentice-Hall, Inc.

Stewart, D., and Stewart, L., editors: Safe alternatives in childbirth, Chapel Hill, N.C., 1976, NAPSAC, Inc.

Ward, C., and Ward, F.: The home birth book, Washington, D.C., 1976, Inscape Publishers.

Wessel, H.: Natural childbirth and the family, New York, 1973, Harper & Row Publishers, Inc.

UNIT IV

Birth experiences

You are about to read a collection of intimacies about birth experiences, as told mostly by the fathers of newborn infants, in the form of conversations, interviews, and photographs. Most of these shared experiences were related to us within minutes, hours, or days after the births.

The majority of these men took time to prepare for childbirth and also for parenthood by actively participating in some kind of childbirth preparation classes.

The fathers whom you are meeting here talk spontaneously about childbirth as they experienced it, expressing what it meant to them to be involved and to share in labor and birth. When asked to share their experiences, all the fathers seemed to enjoy the opportunity to talk about their thoughts and feelings about becoming fathers, even though they often found the experience difficult to describe in words.

As they share with you the wonder, joy, pride, anger, jealousy, insecurity, anxiety, fear, and moments of disappointment and surprise, we hope that you will experience the feeling we had when compiling these accounts—the feeling that these experiences were not an end in themselves but a beginning, a part of a growing, a part of becoming a parent, but perhaps, most important, a part of becoming a father.

"It's 2 days since the baby was born"

Well, here I am. It's 2 days after the baby was born, and I want to tell you a little bit about everything that happened.

I was working when Valerie called me about 11:15 A.M. and told me she had lost her water, that it had broken, so I jumped in the truck and started for home, which is a ½-hour drive. Believe me, it was pretty hectic coming home, trying to go fast, watching for highway patrolmen, and hoping that I'd be there on time because I wanted to be there when the baby was born.

It was exciting. I got all pumped up with adrenaline, came charging home, arrived at the house, changed my clothes, jumped in the car, and headed for the hospital—again all pumped up. Going down the road was really hectic, trying to move as fast and as safely as possible and trying to help Valerie relax during her contractions while I was watching cars, watching speedometer, and trying to time the contractions. We did OK in the car because I told Valerie to tap me on the arm when she had a contraction. When a contraction started, I'd feel a thump on my arm and hear Valerie say, "Battista help me." I had a self-winding watch on, which I hadn't worn for 6 months to a year and the darn thing wouldn't go anywhere even though I kept jiggling it, so I couldn't time the contractions, which is probably just as well, since they were coming very close together and may have scared us to know how close. Well, when I felt the thump on my arm, I tried to help Valerie relax while concentrating on my driving. It was like having to be in twenty places at once and was the most exciting drive of my life.

When we got to the hospital, the lady learned we were preregistered and took us to the OB department after giving Valerie an ID arm band.

In the labor room it was hectic because I was still pumped up with adrenaline and didn't coach Valerie as well as I could have if we'd had an hour of labor at home. If we'd had more of a "warm up" to labor, I could have had time to sit and catch my breath instead of just run, run, run. It was like playing football—trying to catch a guy 20 yards ahead of you and knowing you can never get there, even though you must.

Just 1 hour 36 minutes after Valerie had phoned me at work, our daughter Nicole was born. Even though this was our first baby, when we went to the delivery room, the room wasn't new to us because we had toured the hospital earlier to check it out and see where everything was.

When I scrubbed up to go into the delivery room, I was wondering what it really would be like. A lot of people had told me that the afterbirth and the blood would be nothing, and we had been to a whole series of childbirth classes, but still in the back of my mind was doubt. And there I was, 6 feet tall, 240 pounds, with nurses and a doctor watching, and me worrying about throwing up!

Well, I didn't throw up or faint or any other horrible thing. I was standing by Valerie, rubbing her forehead a bit, because the nurse was controlling her pushing and breathing and helping her, since I was still kind of excited. I watched the baby come out. I feel that if people are going to have children, not because it's the thing to do but because they've talked about it and really want children, the father should be there when the baby is born. It's an experience I'll never forget as our daughter grows up. Just think—when she started out she was as big as a head on a pin, and when she was born, she was 7 pounds 12 ounces, and someday she may be 5 feet 7 inches tall. That's quite a little miracle we have going for us.

When Nicole was coming out, she was a little blue; then when they turned her for her shoulders to come out, she cried a little bit, Waaaa. . ., and her color started to become pink. It was fantastic. They cut the cord, and nothing was a bloody mess like I'd heard from some people who had never been there.

The placenta was like a piece of steak, not gory. It came out shiny side up, and there was a little bit of bleeding but not enough to make me woozy or anything. It was beautiful.

When the baby was lying slanted down in the Kreiselman, she started wriggling out of her blankets so that her head was about to touch the metal bottom of the unit. I called this to the nurse's attention, and she said, "Oh, just pull her up and wrap her." I said, "Whoa, wait a minute!" I didn't want to squeeze her too hard—after all, she was a newborn human and I didn't know how to handle her. Well, now I know I don't have to treat her like a thin glass shell or a bottle of nitroglycerin—I just have to be gentle and careful.

Valerie was in the hospital about 24 hours, maybe a little less, and we brought the baby home. Our life-style has changed so much. It's exciting to hold Nicole and touch her; she doesn't really play now, but she'll wiggle around and open her eyes when I talk to her. It's been fantastic to have a few days off from work to be with my wife and help her around the house and with the baby so she can rest and recuperate.

Today I went down to the store to buy some diapers and a lady saw the box and asked me if I was going to change diapers? "Yes, as soon as she gets a little older," I answered. "The baby's only 2 days old now and really tiny." The lady thought that was great so I told her about being in

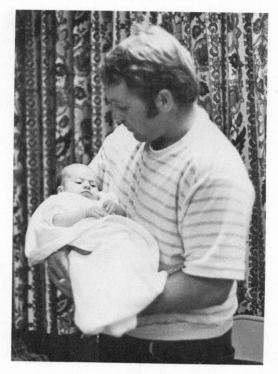

Battista and Nicole.

the delivery room when Nicole was born. She never had that chance and wishes she had. And you know, I wish she and her husband had had the chance, too.

"She's beautiful"

She is just really beautiful—the whole thing was beautiful. She is really good sized with lots of hair and blue eyes, wanting to suck her thumb, shoving her hands in her mouth. I couldn't believe once we got into transition that it was so easy. Sheila went from 3 centimeters to birth within 20 minutes. It was unbelievable once she started to move. I felt helpless to do anything to assist, even though I felt in control the whole time.

I saw the head coming before the doctor got there and thought, "Geez, we are going to go without the doctor." I didn't think he'd make it, but that was OK because I wasn't worried about that at all. The one thing that saved us was the breathing. At one point I forgot the breathing patterns,

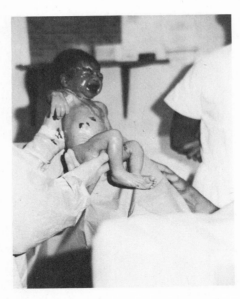

"She's beautiful."

started to lose control, but when I remembered the breathing, it brought us back under control and we were in good shape. It's really something, really beautiful. The head came out and she was born—no waiting at all. She was born immediately. She was on her way, and there was nothing we were going to do about it. She's really beautiful. She really looks so alert, and that's what's unreal to me. I've never been in on a birth before, but that's got to be it, no drugs, and she's just totally awake and already sucking. I can hear her.

I think I knew it was a girl before the doctor because her back was to him and he had to turn her over.

It's funny the thought that flashed through my mind was "Now, I have a daughter to give away at a wedding." It's really funny that went through my mind. She is so beautiful. Here it is 1:20 or 1:30 in the morning.

After the birth of my little baby girl Candice April, the one thing that goes through my mind so often is the fantastic training I received and how the training came in handy when the time was there. It's the one thing Sheila and I both agreed on—without the training there was no way the birth would have been as easily done as it was. The training is absolutely essential, and it happens naturally. But if you know what's happening when it happens, you can remain in control completely and not worry about a thing. Yes, we now have a little baby girl in the family.

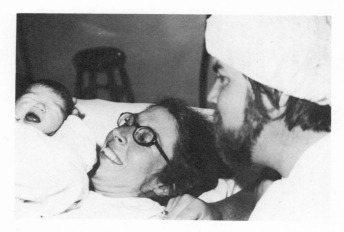

"My wife and my little girl."

Yes, it was a lot of work and a lot of effort on a lot of people's parts—mainly Sheila, and a lot of me, and an awful lot of the nurses and our coach. The beauty of the work is that it came naturally, not easily because it is work, but naturally because we were properly trained.

Right now I'm preparing to go down into town to see my wife and my little baby girl. The doctor has looked at the baby and said she's perfect, perfectly healthy, very alert, and everything works. Sheila is healthy and ready to come home, and I'm going to go down, and we are all going to come back home.

It's only been 17 or 18 hours since the birth of our little girl. Because they received no drugs or anesthetics, my wife and little girl stayed wide awake, alert, not sleepy, and just beautiful.

The doctors have given me the OK, and so the whole family is going to be together today within an hour.

"I've only been a father for 15 minutes"

Lawrence: It's beautiful, Christine was so good. You didn't even need a coach, Christine. You could have done it yourself. I don't know if I can say what it meant to see him born . . .

It didn't look like a head—it looked like a sponge. It's so beautiful.

I was happy it was a boy although I was afraid Christine wasn't because she wanted a girl, but she is happy now.

What does it feel like to be a father? I don't know yet; I've only been one for 15 minutes. I haven't even changed a diaper yet.

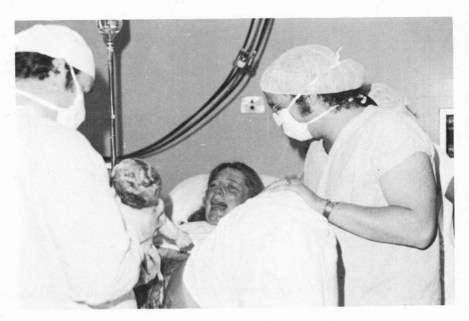

"I had you."

"A conversation"

Lawrence: I've been a father for a day now, and I'm a little more calmed down. It's hard to say how I feel. We are just really happy the baby is here and is healthy and Christine feels good. She did really well during the whole labor and amazed me. I don't think I could have done as well because I would have tired out long, long before the birth.

At one point it seemed like labor would go on forever. I couldn't understand why it was happening so slowly. It wasn't supposed to happen this way. It was supposed to be all easy just like the books, but it wasn't just like the books. It's incredible Christine could hold out for 14 hours. All the credit goes to her.

Christine: No it doesn't—I couldn't have done it without you. You were my strength.

Lawrence: I just don't know how she did it.

Christine: I had you—someone who cared about me and cared about our baby.

"A sharing of private feelings"

Well, I have had very, very strong feelings but don't know how widespread they are, although I have talked to a number of fathers and they identify with the feelings I have. These are feelings of intrusion and maybe a little jealousy, anxiety, and general uptightness about another man working with their own wife in parts that other men normally shouldn't be working with. It's something that came up in very significant terms when we thought of a pregnancy because there are no women OBs in this small county.

Probably many men have feelings like this, but they suppressed them to the point where it doesn't bother them anymore. I think now it's taken care of, probably, but I don't feel in a very helpful, positive way—I've been forced to sublimate like the rest of our guys have according to our culture.

The first thing I would strongly encourage and advise is that we somehow get more female gynecologists. Although when you talk with other women about going to a woman doctor about women's problems, many of them get very uptight about going to a woman. They want to go to a man.

It's possible, as I look back on it now, that it is a self-curing type of thing because as I look back on delivery and labor, I personally was very careful to make sure that either the door was closed or I had a sheet held up when they were working with Sam so that she had privacy. So the modesty thing here—that's a heavy feeling on my part and on Sam's part, too. I was particularly conscious of that all during the process. As a matter of fact, I personally shut the door on the delivery room. They didn't bother to close it. But the one going to the hallway was flopping open and shut all the time so I just walked over and kicked the other shut. No one said anything, and it's probably a good thing. There was no doubt in my mind that that door was going to be shut.

Labor and birth was a neat experience—in fact one of the most fulfilling experiences.

Sam's comment all through the first part of labor was, "Gee, I hope this is real. I expected pain at the top of the uterus, and there is no pain at the top, just a tightening." At 6 centimeters she said, "So you think this is real." She's had 2 hours of 5-minute pains—"Man, 5 minutes plus or minus 10 seconds."

My feelings were that I'm not going to get uptight about this thing and add to any kind of hassle that Sam might have, so I just maintained my cool and said, "Well, if this is for real, then you are going to get some pretty good times on this and you are going to get consistent times. According to the class, false labor is very inconsistent usually." So I decided the best thing for me to do was to get some sleep if I was going to have to be up for 3 days. So I was very selfish and went to sleep.

About 2 o'clock Sam came in and said to look at the times I've got. So I said, "We'd better get hold of the doctor." He said to come to the hospital, so we went—no rush, rush, no runaround. It was easy to stay relaxed. She was into her breathing a long time before I was aware she had a pain at all. So my whole trip was—don't wreck it for her, just keep cool and play it down. But when it came time for action, we took decisive consistent action and showed up at the hospital like the doctor instructed. When the nurse said the cervix was dilated to 3 centimeters, my first thought was, "Well, that's 60 percent of 5 centimeters." We went in really on top of it.

I wanted to maintain a consistency because she was functioning fairly well under that. In fact she was functioning great. Whenever a pain had a peak in the middle, my biggest function was to maintain back pressure and support. My number 1 priority was to get pressure on her back. She came close to losing control twice. I had to move my hand a little as I was in the wrong spot, but as soon as I moved my hand, she got it back together. It felt the rippling of muscles right alongside the spine or right alongside the coccyx as my hand pushed against there. I guess my hands are pretty big so they can reach clear across that whole area, and I could feel that muscle under there ripple back and forth. The ripples were strong enough so that I felt like I could correlate those ripplings with the peaking and the subsiding of her pain.

Yes, I would definitely do this over again—I have strong feelings about people going into childbirth without this kind of preparation. I think it must be one of the most horrendous experiences there is. No, I wasn't scared in the delivery room. I felt confident that my wife was on top of it. I was concerned about that and wanted to keep her up there.

In fact, when the nurses were busy putting her in the stirrups, I was busy pulling up socks on her legs. The two nurses were busy adjusting the table. A contraction came, and I could tell Sam was unsure whether she should push or not. I put one arm under her and raised her up because the delivery table was flat at that point; then she grabbed her knees, and I encouraged her to push. We did that twice while the nurses were getting ready.

Another feeling I had in the delivery room was that we were surrounded by very confident personnel. They knew exactly what was happening. They knew how to do it. They argued that the forceps were labeled as the wrong kind. My wife was on top of it. If I couldn't see, I would just lean over and look.

When my son was born, I didn't have an overwhelming feeling at first. I had a feeling of very reserved exhilaration—I guess it's a thing in our family for men to show no emotion. So I can't really identify any exhilaration or soft-shoe type of thing. I imagine it was there, but it didn't surface. I was extremely pleased and proud of my wife.

I had a definite concern there was not a lot of respiration even after they sucked the baby out. He sort of looked around with one eye, put his hand over his head, turned over, and went to sleep.

"Wait a minute." I thought, "This isn't like they show on TV." But I realized that isn't always right. Then I figured they knew what they were doing, and it was cool, but I'm going to watch that color. So pretty soon comes down the pink color, and he must be getting oxygen some way because that cord is cut. He's turning pink so it's all right.

You know, I ordered a girl for the ninth of May—being a boy was quite a defeat at school and every place else when my order didn't come through. I had to make all kinds of excuses of the stork not being able to get in the window and my wife not being very logical . . . But as I think about it . . . you know . . . a boy is fantastic, man, because there's a guy to go fishing with and a guy to buy a train set for. In fact, today I'm going out to buy him a train set.

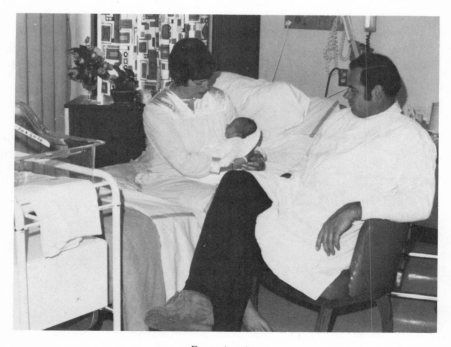

Rooming in.

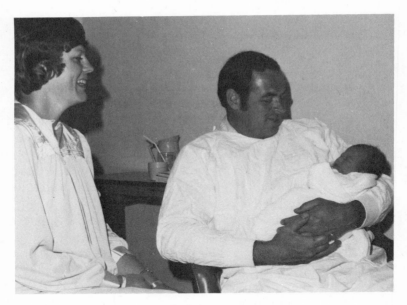

The beginning.

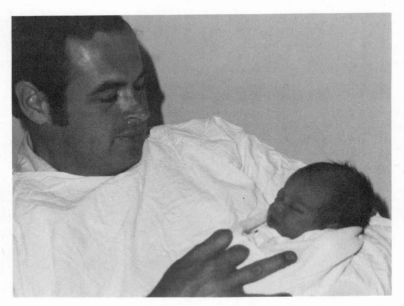

"A guy to buy a train set for."

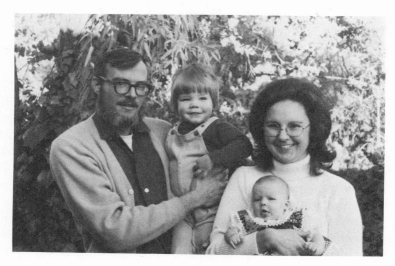

The Vaux family.

"Birth report of Katherine James Vaux"

There were two things that impressed me prior to the birth of our second child. The first was that second labors tend to be shorter than the first, and the second was the fact that during Prindle's first labor she was 5 centimeters dilated before she felt any contractions even worth timing. Additionally, having been through the first labor and delivery, I was extremely anxious to have the baby born at the hospital under the supervision of someone who knew what was going on. I was prepared to deliver the baby myself had the need arisen, but after seeing the difference a trained person can make, even in the face of minor aberrations, I was not at all keen about the possibility that we might not make it to the hospital the second time.

Consequently, when Prindle reported on Monday, September 30, that she was 4 centimeters dilated, I felt that active labor would begin fairly soon. More importantly, I felt that when it did begin, it would be fast. Thus, when Prindle reported early Tuesday morning that she had lost some mucus, I believed that developments were not far off. Given baby-sitting uncertainties and the fact that it could take us as long as 30 minutes to reach the hospital, I felt that I would be more comfortable by staying at home. Moreover, I could see that I would have great trouble concentrating on anything at work for wondering what was going on at home. We had waited so long for this labor to start that I was perhaps more consumed with it than I was willing to admit.

After a futile day of waiting (during which I was lucky enough to get in a 2-hour nap which I needed badly), we went to bed. I slept briefly and apparently fitfully (Prindle said I was talking in my sleep). I was awakened by Prindle rolling over and lay in bed wondering if I would ever get back to sleep. After a few minutes Prindle asked if she could see my watch, and I thought with relief, "Finally some action!" Since my watch is not helpful for timing contractions in the dark, I climbed out of bed, turned on the light, and got the stopwatch. The contractions seemed to be erratic, and I couldn't make much sense out of them in terms of where she might be in her labor.

Suddenly Prindle got up and said she thought she was leaking and felt pressure and went to the bathroom. The previous contractions had lasted 40 seconds and had come at approximately 3-minute intervals. Prindle was doing a little deep chest breathing, which surprised me, since I figured she would go a while without needing to breathe.

I decided that we had better get the decks cleared, called the babysitter, and took our son to her house about a mile away. When I got back and about 10 minutes later, the contractions were 2 minutes apart and lasting about 30 seconds. Prindle told me that my coffee made her feel nauseous and that she felt irritated about my sitting on the bed to time her contractions. As far as I was concerned she was in transition, and I wanted to get going. I persuaded Prindle to call the doctor only after threatening to do it myself. We departed for the hospital after some discussion about what she should wear. (When this question was raised, I really began to believe that I was pushing ahead too fast, since I figured we ought to just go!)

On the way Prindle had three or four contractions and asked me to slow down as they came on because the freeway seemed rough to her and made things more difficult. In the interim I alternated between inquiring of Prindle as to how she felt ("I feel a little pressure") and fantasizing about how I was going to handle the cop who was bound to stop me for some minor infraction.

On arriving at the hospital, Prindle was checked while I, one, paced, two, checked her in after being requested to do so by the nurse, and three, took a tranquilizer. I got into the labor room about the same time as the doctor, who examined and announced 7 centimeters. This didn't impress me much because Prindle was fast panting and we needed to get the bed more upright to make her comfortable. The doctor sat at the other bed and shot the breeze, stopping whenever there was a contraction. At this point

I figured we were going to be there a while. I got Prindle some ice and got set up to time contractions. After what seemed like 3 minutes, Prindle asked for more ice. The doctor said, "No, we have to go." Apparently he was alerted by Prindle's complaints of pressure.

There was really only one potential problem in the delivery room—when she first felt the urge to push, she was very uncertain about what to do. My status was none too hot because the surgeon's mask was fogging my glasses and I felt like I couldn't get any fresh air (I cheated and lifted the bottom of the mask and sucked up!), but I yelled at her to pant-blow. Prindle simply blew, and it worked wonderfully. That was one exercise we had been extremely confident of all along and had been practicing only to keep her proficiency up. The delivery proceeded very smoothly, and we were delighted with our little girl.

In retrospect, I think the ease of the labor was worth waiting for. Despite Prindle's feelings that she never knew where she was in the labor progression, and the consequent anxiety about "prescribing" her breathing, she was on top of it all the way. The one exception was the reminder to pant-blow—that was the only "coaching" I really did aside from attempting to yell up some encouragement. I am convinced that Prindle was in transition almost from the moment she woke up. Her reaction to the coffee and my bed sitting seem to support this. She was definitely in transition in the hospital parking lot, as she was crankily adamant that I not touch her. Prindle looked better and said she felt better 5 minutes after the birth than she had in a month. In actuality there was little reason why she could not have left the hospital and come home then and there.

Finally, I must add that although we broke many hospital rules to do it, the opportunity to have my daughter and feed her a little bit within an hour after birth meant more to me than I can ever say. It was especially nice in that there were just the three of us in a room all to ourselves. I can't see any reason why we couldn't have spent the night in there together. While I recognize that there are situations where this is not advisable, this was not one them. I hope that in the near future our local hospitals will follow the example set by many hospitals in northern California in allowing fathers to be with and to handle their children while they are still in the hospital.

"Prepared childbirth"

Childbirth, as experienced with my three older children during my first marriage, was a nuisance to me and a painful experience for my wife. This was primarily due to old-fashioned traditional ideas and customs.

She missed a period, was sick all the time, and as the months dragged past, she got bigger and more uncomfortable. Finally, after ten months of pain and suffering we traveled to the hospital where I sat in a stuffy waiting room with other men, all of us "miserable expectant fathers." I was worrying about the bills; "How am I going to pay for this whole mess?"

Unfortunately, when my child was born, I felt only relief. Then the journey home to spend the next six months with little sleep and one hell of an adjustment period.

All the above negative feelings are what both my wife and I felt with all of our three children. I believe I felt that way because I was not able to participate in the birth, the labor, or any of the predelivery care. I had little or no knowledge of any of the delivery/birth procedures. If I had been allowed to participate, I would not have known what to do.

When my second wife of only a few months conceived a child, I began having the same negative feelings about the birth experience with one difference—it was more expensive now than nine years ago when my last daughter was born. Then in Charlotte's fifth month of pregnancy, we were invited to participate in a class instructing us in prepared childbirth. My thoughts at the time were, "Why should I do this? I have been through three pregnancies already." It was very easy for me to be apathetic about the whole bloody thing.

When the date for the first class came around, I tried to get out of it. I told Charlotte I was tired, I had had a rough day at work. I wanted to stay home, have a few drinks, and go to bed. But she is a very insistent person, so I gave in and we went to class.

I became interested in what I had learned and the perspective I had gained during that first class. What happened to us during the birth of our son was a result of being prepared for childbirth.

Charlotte and I left for the hospital at 7:00 A.M. The doctor had seen her the day before and decided it was necessary to induce labor for the welfare of the baby. After the preliminaries labor was induced, and contractions started at 8:15. We were ready. As each contraction came, we used the breathing and exercise techniques we were taught and had practiced for the past two months.

When Charlotte reached 5 centimeters, she got stage fright. I knew what phase of labor she was in and could help her. When she reached 6 centimeters, she forgot her lines. Because I was there and could remember what to do, I coached her, calmed her down, told her what to do, and she told me she loved me.

During the labor she wanted to stop, to go home, but the nurses and I

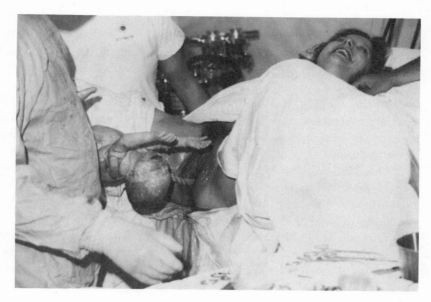

"A moment of joy."

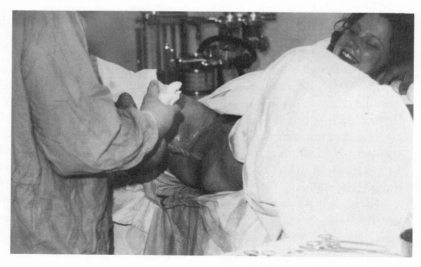

"The most supreme moment."

spurred her on. The nurse came in to check the baby's heart rate, and she couldn't hear it. Without training we would have been frightened and expected problems, but we knew it was because of Charlotte's position, and the heartbeat was finally heard. I reassured Charlotte; I really did something for her and for our baby.

At the very end the doctor, who had been in and out since we arrived at the hospital, came in and gave her a paracervical block. After that small bit of Xylocaine, Charlotte relaxed more and was able to handle the contractions.

Our labor was only 3 hours 1 minute. Christopher Aeron was born at 11:16 A.M. We experienced the most supreme moment a couple could experience. Watching our son pop out of her womb was an experience, a moment of joy I will treasure the rest of my life.

Our son is healthy and happy. I love it all. It is not a nuisance—it is fantastic. I loved my first three and I love Christopher, but I also really like him. I am closer to Charlotte and him as a result of our birth experience.

"It's a whole new life for us"
Mother's story

My labor was how I expected it to be. I didn't realize the importance of relaxation and concentration of your contraction. But it really makes a big difference. A few times I let the contraction get the best of me, and I lost control. It was very painful, but when I relaxed and used my abdominal breathing, it wasn't bad at all.

My husband is the main reason my labor went well. He really gave me a lot of support and kept me from giving up. I couldn't have done it without him. I had a lot of back labor also and so by him rubbing my back, it relieved a lot of the pain.

The delivery was the easiest part for me. It was so exciting I didn't even have any pain. I was pretty lucky and didn't have an episiotomy, so that helped. It felt great to push and what a relief when she came out.

The nursing staff was great. They let me do almost anything the way I wanted to, as long as it was OK with the doctor and not harmful to me. For example, I didn't have a prep or enema, and they didn't strap my legs during the delivery. We were both very pleased with the nursing staff.

Nicole's birth was one of the most precious and meaningful events of my life. I feel it's a beautiful reflection of two people's love for each other. Seeing how much Sam cared for me during the labor and delivery and him holding her so proudly right after she was born made me the happiest person in the world.

Now, it's a whole new life for us. She really adds a lot to both of our lives. It's a lot of work raising a child and a lot of sacrifices, but it's worth it. I wouldn't want it any other way. I feel it's brought us closer, too!

The only thing I would want to change is I wish we could have had more pictures of the delivery and that I could have watched her being born. I forgot to look because I was so busy pushing.

Father's story

I was really excited when Barbara's labor had started, even though it was 3 o'clock in the morning. About 12 hours later I was feeling pretty tired, but I was glad to see that Barbara was able to control herself through her labor, except the couple of times when the contractions had gotten her a little scared.

Nicky's birth was the happiest event that has happened to the both of us. She has only been with us a short while now, and we have been able to see changes both physically and mentally. I also think it's great to be able to take part in the birth of your child and to be there the whole time next to your wife's side. The final moment of birth, to be there, is worth any discomfort that one might go through, through the labor stage.

Barbara and I went to some classes that were conducted by a couple (man and wife). The classes we attended were in an eight-week course which met once a week at the office of the obstetrician whom we had been seeing. The classes helped us understand exactly what was going on during the different stages of Barb's pregnancy.

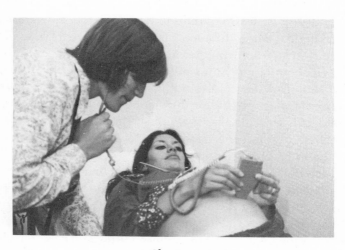

Sharing.

The instructors recommended a book for us to read that was written by Dr. Bradley called, "Husband-Coached Childbirth." Dr. Bradley had interviewed several couples, some of whom had their baby naturally and some who had medicated births. The stories told by medicated mothers sounded pretty scary.

I don't think there would be anything that I would like to change because the staff that was on during our time in the hospital I thought did a really fine job and even shared an interest in Barbara's delivery.

The first night we had Nicole home she seemed to wake up every couple of hours, which was pretty rough on Barbara. The biggest problem the first week I think was too much company, but other than that all three of us adapted quite well to the new change.

Doctor Barry Staley

It was a Saturday afternoon, and we were sitting in the backyard, in the sun, when Joyce mentioned, "I've been having contractions fairly steadily for about one-half hour and am having another one now." I looked at her abdomen. I could see the uterus rising up at that particular time. I looked at my watch. I thought, "This would be a convenient time to have the baby," not feeling nervous at all.

This was our second child. Our first delivery was a thoroughly bad experience. Joyce was having strong contractions when she entered the hospital at that time, and she lost a lot of energy hyperventilating. She hyperventilated to the point where she had tingling in her fingers and almost passed out. It was a bad experience. I felt that I had no control over the situation.

Joyce and I are strong individuals, and we were determined this time to make this labor different. I wanted Joyce to attend the prepared childbirth classes during her first pregnancy, but she didn't express any concern about labor. This time she wanted to learn as much as possible, and I attended the classes without hesitation. I had witnessed several births before our first child but had never been part of the labor scene before. This was all to be new to me. I felt the classes gave us an edge on understanding and the confidence to go through labor in a controlled manner.

After finishing watering the lawn I went in to shave. Joyce took a shower. The contractions were now 5 minutes apart. We both felt that it was time to start for the hospital. We called good friends to come and stay with our daughter. On the way to the hospital I felt concern. I wondered if the baby would have any abnormalities and how our daughter would accept a new child. Most of all, I wondered if Joyce and I would work well together as a team. I knew Joyce had practiced on her own—the breathing and pushing—but together we had only practiced about six times. All of this was very much on my mind. We arrived at the hospital at 3 o'clock. Everything seemed simple—a ride in a wheelchair to the labor area, and then a friendly nurse, Sandy Small, who made us comfortable. We felt we were in good hands. The atmosphere in the hospital was controlled and calm and a very even pace. There was only one other patient in labor; that was very nice.

I started helping Joyce through her contractions. She was breathing just superbly and was on top of it right from the beginning. At this point I felt very confident because I was comparing this to her last labor. When first examined Joyce was 3 centimeters dilated, and in 1½ hours she was 6 centimeters and well effaced. I knew things were progressing fast, and I tried to give Joyce positive reinforcement. The doctor told me that the other patient was progressing along at the same rate—this gave me some anxiety, wondering who would be first to the delivery room.

At 5:15 contractions were pretty strong. The doctor asked Joyce if she wanted a paracervical block. She felt this would be fine, and so it was given. Although she was in complete control throughout, it seemed to help quite a bit. At 5:45 her membranes ruptured, and the doctor told Joyce that she was completely dilated and could now push. In just three contractions with pushing we were ready to go to the delivery room.

The nurse earlier brought me a scrub suit, and now when I went to put it on, I found that there were 2 tops and no bottoms. I had a little anxiety at this point, not wanting to miss the actual birth. I could feel the excitement, but still I was a lot more relaxed than I had been the first time. I was much more pleased with the situation, knowing the end was just around the corner for Joyce and myself—and then with a few more pushes in the delivery room the critter hatched!! It was a tremendous feeling to hear the cry. It was a boy—that was really neat. He was good looking and healthy. It pleased me a lot that he was a boy. It was a tremendous feeling of joy and wonderment in the whole process of life and birth. It was interesting that the fact it was a boy was important— much more important than I thought it would be. A lot of people had asked me if I wanted a boy. I'd say it would be nice just to have a healthy baby. That was my first concern, but being a boy was neat. It was almost the icing on the cake.

The doctor wiped him dry with a towel, waited for the cord to stop pulsating, clamped the cord and handed our son directly to Joyce. She wrapped him in a blanket and held him close to keep him warm. Just looking him over nearly brought tears to my eyes. The nurse asked if I

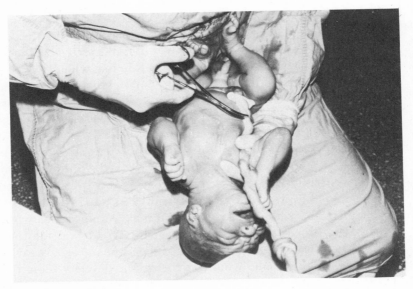

"A boy."

wanted to hold him while Joyce pushed to expel the placenta. I thought, "A woman's work is never really done." The whole thing seemed hard to comprehend—the wonderment of birth itself and the fact that this little crawling thing I was holding was really inside Joyce.

Joyce was helped back to her bed, and we were on our way to Recovery. It was going to be nice to call the relatives and see how pleased they were. I will look back on this with a lot of good memories for years to come.

"My name is Greg Collins"

My name is Greg Collins. My wife Martha and I decided eight or nine months ago, when we were sure she was pregnant, that she would have her child at home, under the supervision of a midwife. The reason for this is not easy to express, but we felt that the hospitals had a certain mystique, not to our liking. If the hospitals would exert a control over the labor and delivery, it would be unacceptable to us. We both felt that we would prefer to deliver at home in a relaxed atmosphere, being as close to the baby as we possibly could, and having with us friends who could share in the birth of our child. I must admit I was very excited and wanted to learn as much about what was going on as I could. I read all the books that I could find about childbirth and prenatal care. We also attended classes to learn breathing techniques that we felt would be helpful in labor.

About 9:30 A.M. Sunday morning, October 13, Martha began having contractions. Her first contractions were not very heavy. It was easy for her to stay on top of this with the use of abdominal breathing. In a couple of hours, however, they began to come closer together, never being more than 2 minutes apart. They stayed pretty much the same all day Sunday, except the contractions seemed to get harder and harder. At 6 P.M. Sunday night we called the midwives. When they arrived, they felt Martha was pretty far along in labor because her contractions were hard, and possibly she was even in transition. We were all really happy and excited and hung out together. She was still having an easy time staying on top of the contractions and was doing panting by then. She hadn't had much to eat, except for some juice to keep her blood sugar up.

Then she started vomiting, which the midwives thought was a good sign because classic transition is accompanied by vomiting and trembling, and having all these symptoms, they figured delivery must be imminent.

Two or three more hours went by, everyone becoming a little bit apprehensive. The midwives did an examination at this point and found that Martha was only 5 centimeters dilated and the baby's head was in a posterior position, which they said would present some difficulty because it would not make good surface to dilate the cervix. They said that she was doing fine, and chances were that if she would just stick in there, she would be able to still have her child at home.

The contractions continued, still coming very hard. She was unable to keep anything on her stomach. We tried all kinds of things—liquids mostly. The space between contractions became shorter and shorter until they were only a minute apart, and they were lasting 45 to 60 seconds. The midwives said they were worried because the fetal heartbeat was up pretty high, which meant the baby wasn't getting as much oxygen as it needed. Martha seemed to be low on energy but decided to stick it out because we felt pretty mutual that if she could just hang in there through the dilatation the baby would turn and be born in a reasonable length of time.

When Martha said she had the feeling that she wanted to bear down, the midwife did another examination and found that she was only 7 centimeters dilated. About midnight Martha started to do pant-blow breathing. I was doing this along with her to help her concentrate, but it just didn't seem she was making any progress. About 4 A.M. an examination showed that Martha was 9 centimeters dilated and the anterior lip of the cervix was swollen and just hanging there. I can't quite picture what that means, but apparently it was preventing full dilatation.

She was still unable to keep any food down and was getting totally exhausted.

Linda and the other midwife decided to phone and ask some other midwives for advice. They said that probably Martha would be in labor another 6 hours. This was a very discouraging prospect. So in view of the fact that the fetal heart tones were so high and Martha's pulse was fast, plus the fact that she was now running a fever and it seemed like things were going to break down unless help was found somehow, we decided it would be a good idea to go to the hospital. We left the house at approximately 7:30 A.M. and got to the hospital at 8 A.M. It was really agonizing for Martha, having these incredibly hard contractions, having to walk down fifty-four steps to reach the car and ride all the way into the hospital.

Once at the hospital, things began happening quickly. The doctor examined Martha, ruptured her membranes, and then with the contractions was able to turn the head with his hand to an anterior position. He said she was completely dilated and could push. An intravenous solution of glucose was prescribed, and I guess gave her a little boost. At 9:39 A.M., only 1½ hours after reaching the hospital, the baby was born. Martha had an episiotomy, a small one, and managed to make it completely through the birth in control and had a natural birth without even a local being used to sew up the episiotomy.

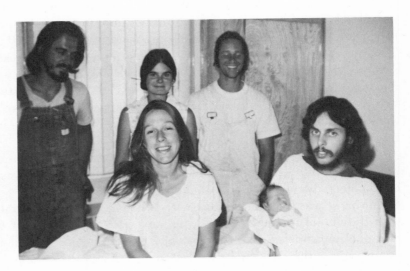

Sharing with friends.

Our feelings about coming to the hospital are very positive. It made the birth experience a beautiful experience for me and Martha, whereas if we had continued on at home things may have been ended tragically. I was really relieved that Martha was able to push the baby out naturally and that she was able to hold the baby shortly after it was born. I was surprised how kind and efficient everyone was, and they respected the fact that we were trying to have our child as naturally as possible. I really have to thank the many friends who were with us at home—there were many things to do for a home delivery, such as boiling instruments, making food for everyone, and even emptying the pail Martha was vomiting in. It is impossible for a husband who is going to coach his wife during labor to be running around and doing all of the other things. Again, I would like to say that the hospital experience was very positive and changed what could have been a nightmare into a really beautiful experience—it was really wonderful.

"So we had twin girls"

Well, it all seemed to begin early on St. Pat's Day, March 17. When I say early, I mean extremely early, because it was 1:50 in the morning when my wife Dorothy came and woke me up and said, "Could you please time my pains? I think I am in labor."

This was theoretically our second child, although actually our third. Dorothy had a miscarriage a few months along, and then we have a 5-year-old son. So you see this was the third one.

We wanted to make sure to get to the hospital on time because the doctor told Dorothy she had been dilated 6 centimeters on Monday, and this was early Wednesday morning. He said he thought it could be any time. We did too.

Dorothy was getting extremely large. We couldn't figure it out because she didn't get nearly that large with our son.

I started timing the pains at about 5 minutes apart, which is when you are supposed to call the doctor, but Dorothy just wasn't sure it was labor because it didn't hurt at all. She could just feel a tightening in her stomach and then it was gone. I felt it, and it felt kind of like a labor pain but I wasn't sure, though, not being an expert at it.

When we had our son, Dorothy had awakened me when her water had broken and I frantically ran around wondering which pair of pants to wear and never did do anything for Dorothy. She had to time the labor and call the doctor. I didn't know what to do. So this time I thought the best thing I could do would be to be calm, cool, and collected and to just help in any way I could. Even so, although I was pretty calm and was timing the pains and helping to call the people where our son was going to stay and helping to call the doctor, it took me three shirts to decide which one to wear. I was still a tad bit nervous, I'd say. We just continued to time the labor pains. They seemed kind of regular, but then they'd get off a little bit. Finally, when it got to 4 minutes apart, we called the doctor and he said we'd better get on in.

We went to the hospital and immediately went to the labor room because Dorothy had preregistered. When we got to the labor room, we told them the pains were 4 minutes apart and not getting 3 minutes apart. They put Dorothy to bed, and the nurse checked her and found she was almost fully dilated at that time and hadn't felt a pain yet. None of them hurt—in fact, she wasn't sure if they were coming or not, and I wasn't either because the timing seemed to be off. The pains were coming, but Dorothy just couldn't feel them. So the nurse told her to tell her when she was having a pain. Dorothy said, "I'm not sure—maybe I'm having one now." The nurse came over and felt it and put the stethoscope on and said Dorothy was definitely having a pain—contraction, that is. Dorothy didn't really feel any of the contractions. This was 3:15—about 1½ hours after she had awakened me.

When we took her into the delivery room, I was able to be there, although I didn't get to talk to Dorothy that much. I would just encourage her and tell her she was doing well. I really didn't know exactly what I was supposed to be doing through the whole thing, since we had only been to two of the childbirth classes.

But it was good, although I felt almost useless trying to be calm, just handle the situation, and bring a stability and security to Dorothy, and that's exactly what happened. She kept telling me afterwards how glad she was I was in there with her. I really didn't do that much—even in the delivery room. All I could do was lift her up when it was time to push and tell her to push. Usually I would just tell her to do what the nurse said to do. I really didn't do very much at all.

But as I've heard people say when they've gone through critical and stressful situations, like the death of a loved one, or just a hard and rough experience, it's not always the people that come over and talk and try to do something with you but it's just the presence of people, knowing that people you really love and care for are present there. So I would say this time that my presence in the delivery room was good for Dorothy in the sense that it gave her security because I was there and we were doing it together. I was involved and could see everything that was going on. They weren't going to get anything past us. We were a team.

So, anyway, in the delivery room Dorothy was pushing and had to pant a few times, and it hurt a little and I could see that pain. I guess that was good for me because I could see what she had to go through in childbirth—you know, I helped cause that. It gave me a greater appreciation of our children and for her. Just seeing the pain and effort she had to go through, even though I didn't get to help a lot, made me hurt for her, and that was good. When you can hurt together, go through pain together, it brings you closer together. It's one of those milestones you can look back on in your marriage and say, "Hey, we did it together." That was a valuable time for me.

So finally the doctor said, "Well, Dorothy one last push and the baby will be out." Dorothy just couldn't believe it, and she said, "Oh! is that right?" She was exhausted and elated at the same time. Then she gave the one last big push, and this baby came out—just a little girl, a red little girl, and a tiny little girl. I couldn't believe how tiny she was because Dorothy was so big, and so as the doctor had her out and handed her to the nurse, he said one of the most unbelievable things I had ever heard. He said, "Oh! there's another one in there." And so we had twin girls!

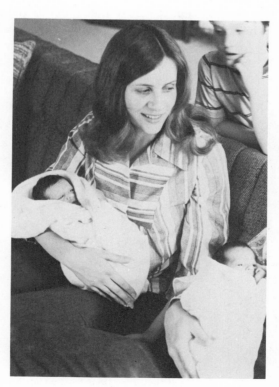

"We had twin girls."

The second one came out feet first and was rather blue when she came out, causing a little bit of concern. Dorothy didn't really understand what was going on the whole time. When the doctor said there was another one coming out, I said, "Are you kidding??" It was just kind of a funny experience . . . and Dorothy didn't really understand, at first, but finally she realized and gave a few more pushes for that second one. It was good for me to be there; I could explain to her that we had twins, and I could help.

Also, I don't think the staff could make Dorothy understand what was happening as well as I could because of the pain she was going through. Also, I could find out how the babies were doing and take that burden off Dorothy. I think she appreciated that.

So we had twin girls—Heather Mae was born at 4:36, and Dawn Michele was born at 4:40. And it was a complete surprise but a good surprise. I have to say I saw those girls come out, and I saw them cut the umbilical cords. I saw them wash them up, put them on oxygen, and I was right there. I have to say it was a smoother transition when we took them home because I was in the delivery room—because I was there all the time. It was consistent for me to take them home, and to help there. I was less hesitant and fearful in helping than I was when I took my son

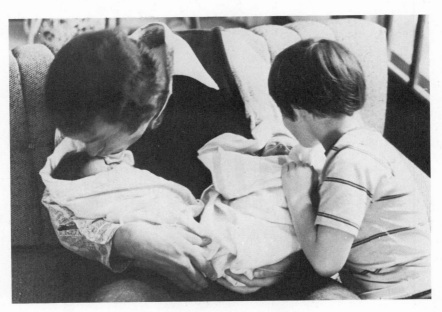

"Children are a gift from God."

home. I don't know if I feel any closer to them than I do to my son, but there was more of a consistent transition when I got home because I was with them. I was there, and also I got to hold them in the hospital, and that made a real difference.

So we took the girls home even though they were very small—4 pounds 14 ounces and 4 pounds 13 ounces.

It's exciting and a great experience to see a new birth. I'm just glad I was able to go through it with my wife.

In the Living Bible it says this about children: "Children are a gift from God. They are his reward. Children born to a young man are like sharp arrows to defend him. Happy is the man who has his quiver full of them. That man shall have help. The help he needs when arguing with his enemies."

Well, children are a great gift from God. They are a reward, and I am happy that I was able to see my quiver filled with two more . . . and I'm glad I was able to see the whole thing.

"There's a closeness now"

I think I can kind of understand why the population is what it is in the world. This is my second birth. It's getting better as it goes. Our first child is a little boy, 3 years old, and I was in the delivery room with him when he was born. The birth itself was really nice. The labor wasn't too good because we didn't really understand what was in front of us. It was only good once it got behind us. But as far as the birth went, I really liked being there and watching my child from the minute he took his first breath of air. Maybe he will see me go out the same way. It was something special to me.

This second baby that we had today was really super. Everything was controlled, and even labor was good. It was really nice—I don't know how to express it best. It's nice to see that fathers are getting more into the birth thing than they have in the past. You don't see the husbands' waiting room so full. I think it's partly the husband's job as much as the wife's job to have the baby. It's really nice to see all the proud fathers standing out looking in the nursery window and to be one of them. If all couples can get involved in their birth experiences, it might make the world a little better place and we could start caring a little bit because we all pitched in and worked together to create it.

I feel really privileged to be able to have been a part of the birth, and I think if we ever have another one, I might try to deliver it . . . it probably won't happen because we probably won't have another one, but I would like to get involved in something like that. I really think I could do it and

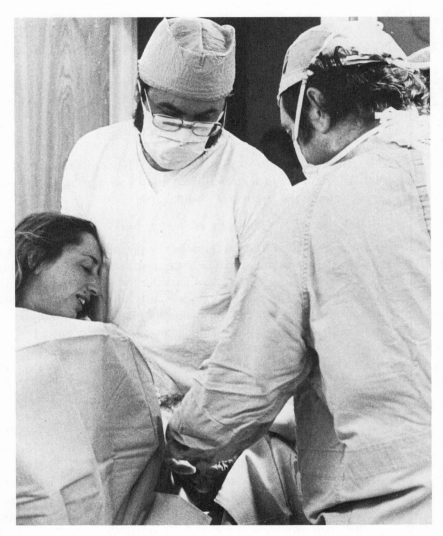

"There's a closeness now."

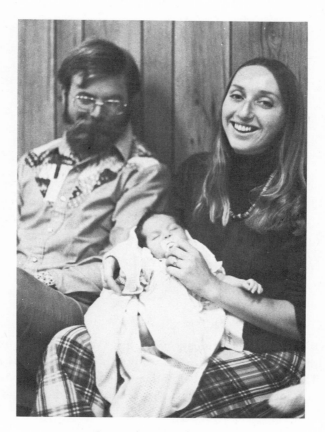

Peder, Lynn, and baby Sommer.

could handle it. I don't think it's all gory and messy like everybody says. It's nice. It's one of those things in life that has to be, and everyone should understand it.

Seeing someone work—that made me feel I had to do what I could to help her. I would have taken half the pain if I could, but that's impossible. My stomach was grumbling as it was anyway, with a full case of sympathy pains.

I feel that after a birth like this, I'm closer to my wife. There's a closeness now that there wasn't before—some understanding.

There's a closeness. . . .

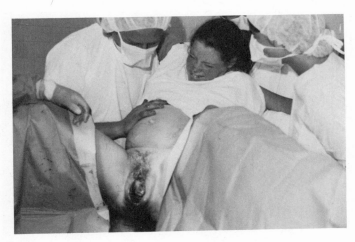

"I started pushing."

"Jaramie"

My labor was induced with an IV slowly dripping. From the beginning the contractions were about 2 minutes apart and 30 seconds long. They seemed to start at both sides of the uterus (about where the hip bones are located), work their way to the center bottom of the uterus, and then work slowly up to the top.

After about 7 hours I felt like I had to go the bathroom. I had a bedpan under me so I sat up to go, and pushed, and realized a contraction had started. (I guess that's what they call "the urge to push.") The nurse told me not to push, but I didn't even realize I was going to push until I was already pushing. Trying to stop pushing was hard and uncomfortable. In fact, I think trying not to push was the only real discomfort I can remember.

When the doctor told me to go ahead and push when I felt like it, I started pushing until the head and one arm was out. Alan kept telling me to open my eyes and see the baby. When I stopped pushing, I opened my eyes. I saw the baby's head and one arm was out. Then as I watched, the other arm came out, then the rest of his body. The doctor cut the cord, dried him, and put him in a towel, and set him on my stomach while he delivered the placenta. Alan wanted to hold him, so I told him to pick him up. He did, and then the nurse asked what we were going to name him. Alan told her, "Jaramie."

In the recovery room I nursed Jaramie for about 20 minutes before he

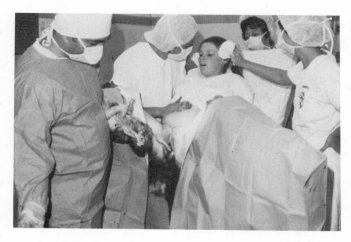

"Stopped pushing and opened my eyes."

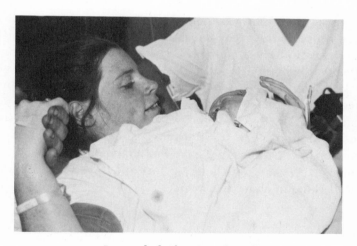

I was glad Alan was there."

was taken to the nursery. I thought the nurses were very nice; they helped us do the things we were taught in class even though it was all very new to them.

I think everything happened about how I expected, but I will say that I expected to feel pain of some kind throughout the whole experience, and I can honestly say the only discomfort I felt was pressure on the bladder and not being able to push when I wanted to.

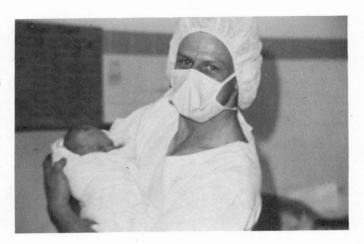

Alan and Jaramie.

I was glad Alan was there. I think since you need both of you to get pregnant, it is only right you should also share the work and enjoyment of delivering it. I know we both enjoyed it, and I wouldn't want to do it any other way. The emotion that fills the room when the baby is born is meant to be shared between both of the parents. I know that his being there made him feel closer to Jaramie and me and has helped to make us happy together. Also the husband knows all that goes on, so he is more understanding when it's time to go home. I think this was the most wonderful experience we have had together in the whole four years of marriage. We are both looking forward to the next child. We plan on another one in about two years.

"It was a painstaking experience"

My name is Bill Costa. When I found out that my wife was pregnant, I went into mild shock. Pauline's first pregnancy had been a problem—partial placenta previa, separation of the placenta, and then premature birth at 7½ months, with the infant's lungs not formed enough for her to live. The baby died 2 days after birth. Because of this, I was very much afraid and didn't know if I was equipped mentally to handle anything that might go wrong with this pregnancy.

We had tried ever since the death of our first baby to conceive again. Finally, in September, my wife went to see the doctor who performed a fertility test and told her she wasn't ovulating, and she had to take fertility pills. She took this medicine during December and January and this month, and then when she went to our family doctor for her annual examination, she was told that she was pregnant.

Let me say one thing—life with my wife being pregnant wasn't easy. For no reason pregnant women seem to be from one extreme to the other—irritable, crying, joyful—but the love you hold for each other and for the unborn infant makes it all right, even if you get uptight at times.

Everything seemed to progress along normally and naturally until about five weeks before the baby was due. I was at work when Pauline called and said that she was bleeding. I drove home immediately, very much afraid, past memories running through my head. Between praying and running through stop lights and traffic, I thought, why us, and why the child? When we arrived at the doctor's office, he examined Pauline and ordered complete bed rest in the hospital. A picture of the baby was taken in the hospital, called an ultrasound scan, showing the baby to be lying crosswise with the placenta in front of the baby. Her bleeding slowed down to just spotting after 2 days of bed rest. Four days later, however, the bleeding started up heavily, this time with clots. The doctors told us that because of this heavy bleeding, placenta previa, and the infant lying crosswise, a cesarean section would have to be done.

As they took Pauline to the operating room, she seemed to be in good spirits, but I was anxious and lonely. I waited, wondering what was happening. It was a painstaking experience that seemed like an eternity. It was the pediatrician who brought our baby, a boy, into the father's waiting room for me to see.

Pauline is now at home. Emotionally, she is glad to be there. I still spend a lot of time helping her as she tires very easily.

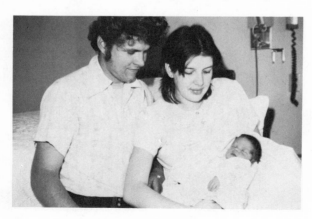

The Costa family.

I must say that it was all a very frightening experience, particularly wondering what was going to happen next, but with all of my trust in the good Lord, as well as the fine people who gave us moral support, everything worked out well.

"About Nathan's birth"

When I left the delivery room, I felt a surge of relief—relief that it was over and Cynthia and the baby were OK. Sometimes during the labor I was frustrated and angry. We told the doctor that we didn't want any drugs, and he told us that he didn't give drugs unless they were needed. Then when Cynthia was complaining of fatigue, he gave her a paracervical block. It seemed to stop the labor for a little while and really stopped her urge to push. This made me angry, although Cynthia seemed relieved and happy to get a rest from the contractions. I guess at that point I just wanted the labor over with, and anything that interfered with its progress bothered me.

Sometimes I think that men have no place telling a woman in labor how to deal with the contractions. It would be better to have more women

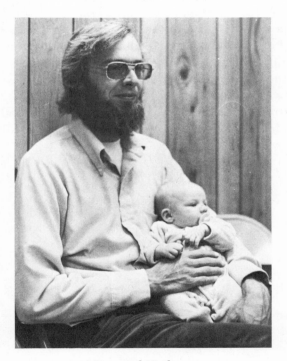

Don and Nathan.

obstetricians or midwives. They would know from their own experiences that a woman may be making more noise and protesting more than she is actually experiencing pain. A woman could reassure another woman that labor would be over soon, instead of offering drugs. It seemed that the doctor just couldn't stand by and watch Cynthia complain of pain and not do something to relieve it . . . instead of just reassuring her and waiting it out. Also, I think that the most important male present should be the father. After all, this was the birth of our son, not the doctor's.

Ideally, the mother, child, and father are the most important because the birth means so much to the family, whereas the doctor will go on to deliver more babies. The husband shouldn't be made to feel like an intruding appendage.

During the hardest part of her labor, I wondered if it was really worth it to have children if Cynthia had to be in such discomfort. It's not easy to stand by watching and encouraging and trying to help the most important woman in your life when she is experiencing fatigue and pain. You see Cynthia had been in labor a long time, and she was tired . . . and so was I. Anyway, we have a great son named Nathan, and he is the result of all our hard work, and he is worth every minute of it.

The labor and delivery weren't all perfect, as I've told you, but I was there and we have these memories to share and talk about the rest of our lives. And maybe when Nathan's wife gives birth, the frustrations that I felt, he will not have to feel because there will be the changes that I would like to see. And he will be the most important man present, and then he will talk to us about it, and we will have come full circle . . . we fathers.

"You are really your own man"

We went into this pregnancy very happy. The baby was wanted; the baby was not an accident.

I think the first time I realized I was getting into hot water was when my wife wanted to go to the classes and I didn't want to go. My feelings toward it weren't running very psychologically deep. It was the fact that I felt I was in a woman's world. I told her it was exactly like going into buy a bra—you know, just not your domain. But I would never have let her go alone. We would have either done it together or not done it. So my wife went to the doctor and asked him about the classes, and his counsel was, "Well, take a look and if you don't want to go to classes, fine." That seemed honest enough, and we both attended every class.

I think probably the greatest psychological help was familiarity. I mean we went to the hospital and saw the labor room and all that stuff. I think the most horrible thing that could have happened would be to have entered that hospital for the first time when the baby was due. That would have been just like moving into the gas chamber. But we had been running in and out of the place so often by delivery time that it was like old home week.

So when D Day arrived, we went in to the hospital and we got her set, expected a full 5 minutes before the show began, but nothing happened and the hours droned by. We waited patiently. Kathy was going through all the normal breathing patterns and they distracted her some, which was fine.

We ground through the first shift and thought they were the greatest thing and were surprised to see that we were still there for the second shift. By then despondency was starting to sink in a little, and Kathy was getting discouraged. We had my daughter coming to visit us quite a bit. She's a comedienne type, and that was a help.

Then night arrived, and the sun went down again, and things ground on. Kathy's problem then was that she dilated to about 6 centimeters and quit—just shut down the show and stopped. Fatigue was beginning to get all of us. I think I was a lot more frightened than Kathy knew. But the complete familiarity of knowing why this was done, why that was done, and we can do this, and we will do this if that happens, reassured me. I had lots of time to think and really, really dreaded the delivery room because I am really a very squeamish person. I could see myself in there totaling out.

Then it got to where Kathy was getting really tired, and the doctor was getting concerned. I figured it would be a cesarean, and I felt really bad because I felt Kathy got the worst of everything. If she went that far without the baby and had the recovery part of the cesarean—she just got gypped in both.

Finally, when the doctor came in, he said, "Well, I think we can go now." But I could just see her pooping out, and I know he could too. When they wheeled her into the delivery room, I couldn't help thinking at that moment the period I was really dreading was that delivery room, but by that time I was leading the charge. I couldn't get in there fast enough. The delivery room was really fun. Really I liked that! By then it just came . . . wow! Bam! I think it was 3 or 4 minutes. I was right there when the baby was right there, too—really it was nose to nose. It was something I'll never forget. I remember thinking that it never crossed my mind it was a girl. I just thought, "My God, it couldn't be. He was too huge." He was 10 pounds 11 ounces. There was this big horse lying there. I remember he was so messed up. His head was just like he had a dunce cap, it was so elongated, but he had this sweet little face, with this ding-dong head. The doctor started stitching Kathy up; he really had a lot of work to do. She was oblivious of this whole thing. I could see so much more than she could. I really had the box-office seat.

I remember the classic thing was that we found out he had toes and fingers. Then what Kathy was trying to say was he's really neat, but what a weird head. She said, "His head is a little strange looking." Boy, it really did look strange. But the doctor said, "Well, buy him a hat." By the next day his head was fine. I think it was so important to be able to get that very first glimpse of him.

When I saw Kathy was OK, I felt really unnecessary. At that point it was the only time I felt that way and wondered, "What am I doing here?" Then later they cut the cord and dumped him in that little table, and he was all by himself, and I remember walking over to him and thinking, "You are really your own man." That was the biggest thrill because he was all unhooked. There he was, a little person all by himself. That face

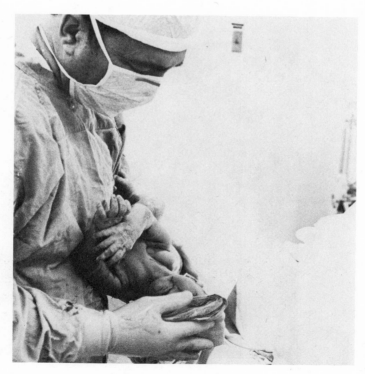

"The boy was right there."

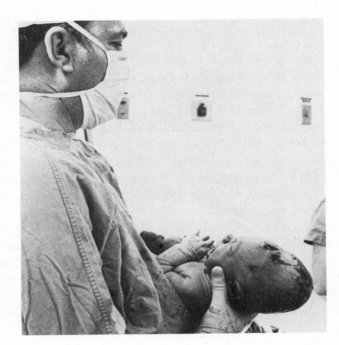

"His head is a little strange looking."

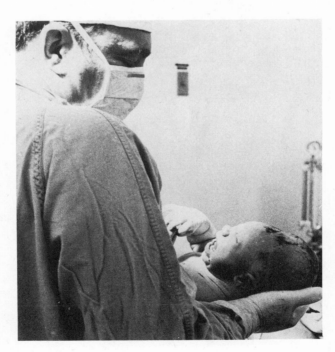

"Buy him a hat."

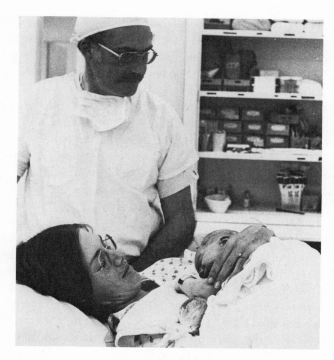

"Kathy and I have shared an experience."

when he first emerged was just this awful look of indignation—like you had just wakened someone at 3 o'clock in the morning. But he took it all in such good stride. I thought to myself, "I really like that guy." You know, I instinctively knew his personality from the time he was 2 minutes old.

Kathy and I have really shared an experience, and I like that feeling. But I think Willy and I have too, and that's really nifty. That's kind of an unexpected dividend.

"It's an active, giving process"

Although I felt very positive about the childbirth classes we attended, I did feel that fathers should have something specific to take to the hospital with them. After all, mothers were given a list of what to take with them. When we went to the hospital, I felt that I needed something for me, so I got a lollipop just for me and even wondered what else I could take. Later on, I ended up borrowing some playing cards and buying a newspaper.

After arriving at the hospital, there was a brief period of time while Sharon was getting prepped that I ended up in a waiting room. I noticed a very positive bonding thing between myself and other people waiting there for babies to be born. People tended to be very friendly, warm, and open about themselves, and it was kind of nice.

When I went back in the labor room and found Sharon was only in very early labor, I felt a certain amount of anxiety and, "Whoops, we're here too early." This caused me embarrassment because the doctor had come in to the hospital on a night when he wasn't really on call. Also, there were a lot of people in very active labor, and all the beds were full. I actually felt a bit guilty for Sharon occupying a bed that maybe we didn't need.

As the hours went by in the night, the embarrassment turned to displeasure that stronger contractions didn't come—to the point where I ended up reading the paper and not talking to her too much. I was really tired then. Sharon looked a lot better than I did, but then she was in bed and I wasn't. At that point a couple of things came to me. I realized that we had practiced the breathing patterns in bed, and the urge to climb into bed with her made me realize that there must be a reason those labor beds are so small! If the labor beds were larger, there would probably be more husbands in them. Even though I knew that this was inappropriate behavior, if things could be different, it would be neat to have a bigger labor bed. It would be much better than sitting across the room in an uncomfortable chair, feeling very tired.

Someone offered me a place to sleep, probably because I was a doctor, so I slept for a few hours in the doctor's lounge. When I returned to the labor room, Sharon wasn't doing any more than earlier, so I went off to do some errands that needed to be done.

When I got back to the hospital, a short time later, Sharon's membranes had been ruptured. This meant that we were committed to having that baby that day, and my feeling that I should know better than to get to the hospital too early felt better. I felt good at that time.

Sharon was looking pretty good, and that really made me involved. Now I had something to do. What was nice was that I wasn't told at a certain time in labor, as I was six years ago, "Well, it's time for you to leave now. We're going to take over. Wait out there, and we'll let you know what happens."

Finally, when things started picking up and Sharon was 5 to 6 centimeters, she was finding out that slow breathing wasn't helpful enough. For the last 2 hours, when the contractions were strong and forceful, we worked together. I felt like I was valuable—doing something. Sharon hurt and seemed to have the feeling, "Stop the world, I want to get off." It was sort of a psychological awareness that it hurt more than she could control and that maybe she was a failure.

My own reaction was, "Well, my God. I know it hurts. But don't worry about it, you're in enough control. It's going to be cool." I felt like I had something to do and did what I could by coaching her, reminding her to keep her eyes open, to breathe, and all this helped. It was a head trip to know all the time that, according to her history, when Sharon went into active labor, she really went fast. So I encouraged her to hold on and not take any drugs. Although I thought if it were me, I'd take anything they offered. And I think this decision in the end made her feel a whole lot better. Sharon wasn't really asking me whether or not to take pain medicine—she just wanted reassurance that she could work through this labor.

Somewhere between 8 and 10 centimeters Sharon said, "I've got to push," and immediately assumed the pushing position. Then I realized, "My God, this is it." As all this happened, I think I would have felt powerless if we hadn't been prepared for changes in moods and feelings. When at last we were in the delivery room, I felt like I had a role because each time Sharon had to push I could support her back and help her by reminding her how to push. The doctor did a pudendal block and put on forceps so the baby could crown. Then it took about three contractions, and without an episiotomy she was born.

Throughout medical school and internship, delivering a baby was just about the most phenomenal and wonderful experience I had. It always fascinated me. But to be there and have my own child was just overwhelming. The experience was excitement and fatigue and happiness in a way I've never felt before. I couldn't quit crying. There had been some wish for a boy, and I'm not sure that recognition that the baby girl led to any disappointment. I remember Sharon saying that she had wished for a boy with our first baby and felt about 10 seconds of disappointment when she saw the girl. Maybe I felt 5 seconds. That's all.

I think the main reason I didn't want to be in the delivery room before, even if it had been offered to me, was because I worried about anoxia, respiratory distress, and what if the baby is malformed? In the past I felt that I didn't want a part of that—that I would be too anxious to deal with it. Having that anxiety removed immediately by seeing that the baby was fine added to my tears of joy. Of course, Sharon felt immediately better as soon as the head was born.

I helped Sharon support the baby on her chest in the delivery room.

Then I held her again and carried her to the recovery room, feeling a warm glow . . . a continuance of the first feeling. I couldn't talk. I was speechless.

When we had seen the pictures and movies of a mother putting the child to breast on the delivery table, I thought it was stylish and plastic. But all of those reservations disappeared when Sharon nursed her. It was, "Wow, look at her nursing!"

It seemed so alien to me that the baby would be with us after just being born. All my past training and experience had been that the mother, father, and baby go their own separate ways. But, my God, here we were all three together.

Next we got on the phone and called the neighbors who had our little girl and said, "Hilary, your sister would like to talk with you." This was another time when I felt overwhelmed and had tears, saying something simple like, "You'll get to see her tomorrow." Joy and tears were all mixed together.

It's almost 24 hours to the minute since Nicole was born, and I'm still feeling like it was a treat, or a privilege, or a gift to be there throughout the whole thing. It's so different to say, "Hello, how are you feeling? Hi, Baby!" as they are being wheeled down the hall after going through

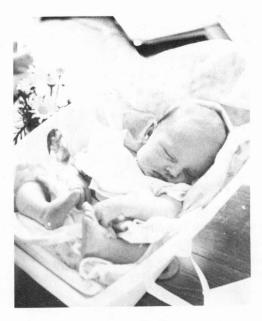

"Hi, Baby."

something in the other room that you were not a part of, all the way. Indeed, it's the difference between having the baby and being delivered. It's an active giving process.

I feel so much closer to my wife. The bond is there.

"Now I believe it"

Suzanne and the doctor thought the baby would be here June 2. When all of a sudden it happened in April, we weren't ready psychologically.

Actually, we had just come back from a short, restful few days in Yosemite when Suzanne went in for an examination because she felt she may have dilated a little more. She's very sensitive to how she feels.

So after her visit to the doctor's office, Suzanne phoned to tell me that she was 3 centimeters' dilated and I had better not go on the out-of-town trip I had planned. I was in a meeting when she called the first time, and then she called me back about an hour later. I asked if she had any labor contractions, and she said, "No, not yet." However, I felt something different, just sensed something, so I stopped by the hospital on my way home and preregistered for us. Then I stopped by the camera store and bought some film and got home about 1 o'clock. We put our son down for a nap and sat down and talked. We just sat there and talked about it, about what might happen, about what to do, and we made sure we had gone down our checklist and were prepared if anything should happen.

We checked on what we thought were false labor contractions because they weren't hard all over but just on one side and not the other. We had a hard time telling whether or not they were real contractions. The first hard contraction was about 3:27 P.M. From that time it was about 2 hours and 32 minutes when the baby was born.

It's still a surprise. It hasn't hit me yet because I was prepared for weeks from now.

I was surprised to see the baby crowning. It seemed we were in the hospital only 10 minutes. I was having a hard time getting these paper shoes on over my shoes, and then I raced to get washed up and go into the delivery room. I couldn't keep up with Suzanne. It went so fast. My first reaction when the baby came out was, "It's a boy!"

I had been really curious as to what we were going to have. My second reaction was, "Baby looks very healthy . . . that's good . . . nicely formed, no apparent problems. See it breathing. A well and healthy baby." It's a good feeling. I never doubted that feeling either that we would have a healthy baby in one piece. If you take care of yourself and think right about it and don't have any genetic history of troubles, there shouldn't be any problems.

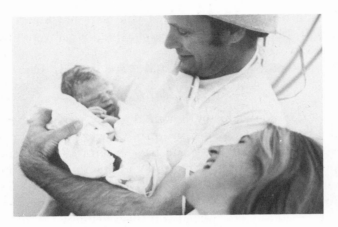

"Now I believe it."

I would have preferred a girl, but I'm not disappointed. I'm sure I will love him as much as I do Steven. He has a wonderful mother, so he will turn out fine.

He's here. He's warm. I can touch him, and now I believe it.

"He was so warm"

When I was a boy, I had a mom who was an R.N., and she gave me some insight into this whole life-birth thing.

Actually, my mom has a great deal to do with my feelings now. She always said, "Michael when you get married, try to have a great deal in common with your wife. Share with her. Do with her." That's not easy for me because I love my photography and could work 80 hours a week.

We've been married four years but have been apart twice in those four years. As a matter of fact when I found out about this pregnancy, we were living apart. Roberta called me up one night and said, "Michael, let's go out to dinner. I want to talk to you about something." Then she said, "It's time to crack that bottle of wine." Well, I knew immediately what she was talking about because I had a bottle of 1957 elderberry wine which my grandmother gave to me when I went away to school. I had told my grandmother that I would not crack that bottle of wine until she was a great-grandmother. So you see, I knew immediately what Roberta was talking about, and I was really happy. However, we still weren't sure how we were going to handle this situation. I needed my own space still and wasn't sure about a lot of things. I was waiting tables, working in

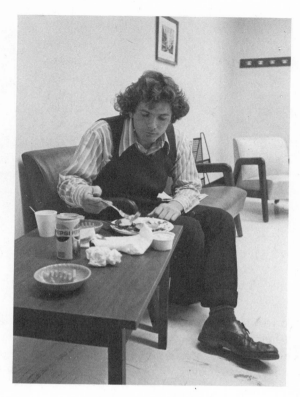

Dinner for a waiting dad.

construction, and trying to develop my photography. Yet I knew this was her child and my child, and somehow I wanted it to work.

The biggest thing I had to do was set aside Tuesday nights for my wife and that growing stomach. We went to preparation-for-pregnancy classes together.

The reaction of my friends was noncommittal: "Maybe it will work; maybe it won't." After the first class I began to relax. It took the class to teach me the role, not to give me my enthusiasm. I felt enthusiastic from the beginning.

As time went on, I quit my construction job, was laid off at the restaurant, and had no job but my photography. I prayed, and I wrote, and I kept a journal. It was then that I decided I wanted to be a photographer and opened up my shop. Somewhere in there Roberta and I decided to go back together again.

As Roberta's tummy grew larger, the wondering grew harder. Bed was

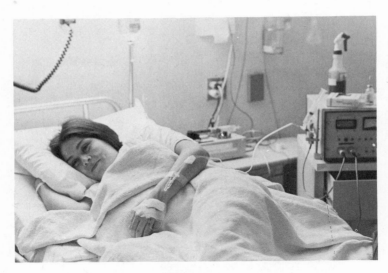

Monitored.

always a good time because we could sit there and talk about it. With lovemaking there were different positions we had to work out; certain positions work out better. Probably, the biggest thing, though, was when the baby first started to move—Boom! Boom! . . . that little kick. It was so great to feel it.

One day I came home, and Roberta had a lot of back pain all Saturday night and Sunday. So we went into the hospital about 5 o'clock Sunday night. Little did we know that the baby wouldn't be born until 7 o'clock in the morning.

They made me wait outside while they admitted Roberta, which really irritated the hell out of me. After all, what were they going to do to her? Shave her, or whatever . . . simple little things . . . nothing I hadn't seen before.

The first thing they did was strap the monitor on her, so we got to watch the contractions.

Nothing was really happening. Roberta was at 3 centimeters and didn't go to 4 centimeters until 2 A.M. Her progress was slow, and it got to the point where she wondered if she would dilate. I read my newspaper. That's another thing—you think you're going to go in there and everything will happen. But it doesn't. It's patience, lady.

Once we got into Roberta's hard labor, the contractions were very hard, every minute. After it got hard, we didn't need the monitor because we just knew when the contractions were coming.

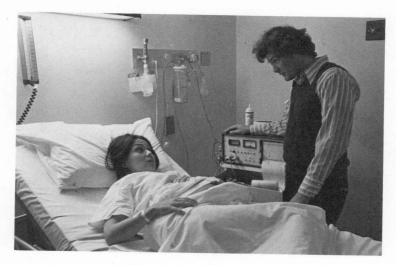

"An innocent bystander."

At times when I couldn't do anything I felt like an "innocent bystander." At times I felt helpless. In spite of this, it was comforting to me to know I was helping her by being there and doing little things, and she would let me know I was helping her.

When we were ready for the baby to be born, it went so fast. By 6:15 she was ready to push. With the first push I saw some forehead, and I said, "Oooh, it's going to happen." They had me get dressed with my boots and everything. I said, "Let me get in there; it's going to happen." I didn't feel good in the delivery room, I know that. That's because they said, "You stand there." I didn't want to because I wanted to photograph my baby's birth. But they wouldn't let me; they said I'd contaminate everything. I didn't want to upset my wife because our baby was going to be born. Therefore I stood where they told me to.

We had gone through all these classes, then the doctor brought out forceps. They looked like huge salad tongs . . . Then Roberta and I said, "Time out." Roberta asked, "Michael, should I have them?" The doctor explained why we needed them then, so we said OK. Then the doctor turned the head and whoosh, he was there.

I've never been higher, elated . . . an exhilarating feeling. I've always excelled with everything—in sports, in school—those are all small achievements. But when that kid comes . . . Wow! That's satisfying. I was also at peace. It's strange. I was as high as a kite for a week. The thing I remember most is I held him right after he popped out, and he was

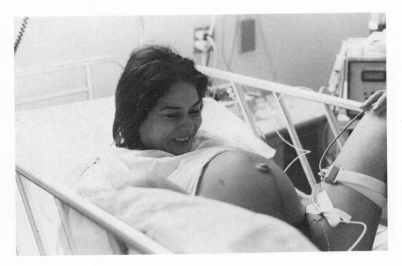

Pushing.

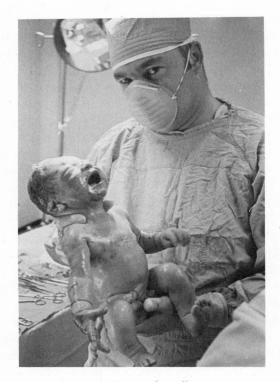

"He was there."

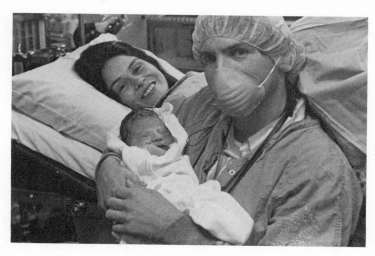

"He was so warm."

covered with a little receiving blanket, and he was so warm. I had to be the proudest man walking the face of the earth.

We were working on this communication before in our marriage, but since the birth, it's been so much better. We used to go to bed and share the events of the day, and as I said, it was a mystery, and we'd just share the mystery, and we share a lot more now.

I can definitely go back to this little baby, and that was a point of departure. Everything is much better for us now.

"The greatest experience in the world"

This was the first birth for both of us, and we both greatly enjoyed the experience. Both of us attended childbirth classes, which really got me, as a "to-be father," interested in childbirth.

During the class we both decided on having an unmedicated birth. Labor for us started at 1:30 A.M. We worked at home with the contractions until 7:30 A.M. Then we called the doctor, I explained what was happening, and he told us to go to the hospital. When we arrived at the hospital, we both got down to work with contractions right away. Sue was 5 centimeters on arrival. Within 1½ hours we were pushing our way to birth.

We delivered a baby girl at 10:12 A.M. Words cannot express the way I

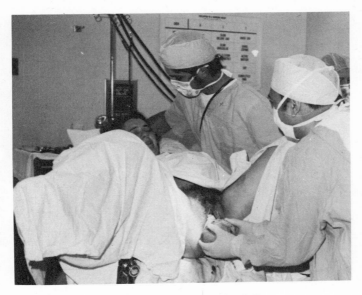

"Pushing our way to birth."

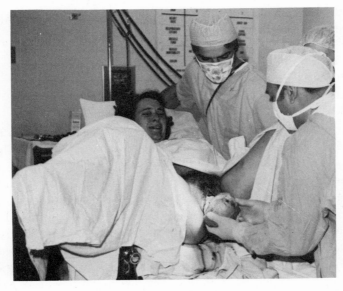

"We delivered a baby girl."

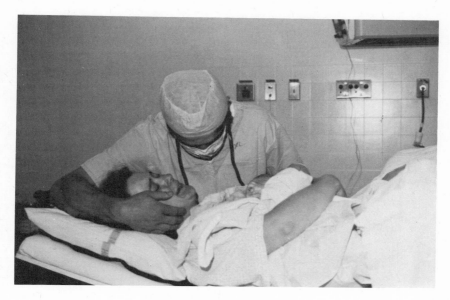

"All I could do was cry."

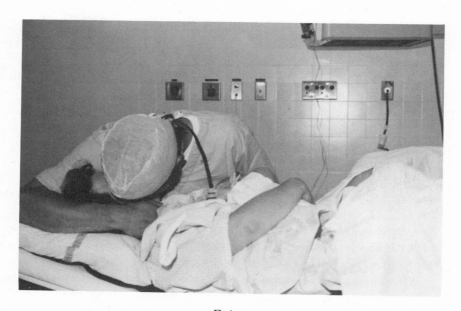

Enjoy.

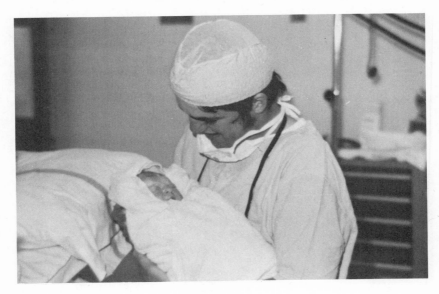

"Greatest experience."

felt in the delivery room. All I could do was cry with Sue and take pictures and enjoy.

Sue was very well relaxed throughout all labor, and I love her for it. When we decide on our next baby, we will definitely prepare for delivery in the same way. It is the greatest experience in the world, and I also urge to-be fathers to attend class and involve themselves in the birth of their child.

"This made me a father"

Little Kurt is our first child, and so far, the entire experience has been so grand that our next has already been discussed.

Sharon learned from the doctor one week prior to the due date that she was 3 centimeters dilated, and she was told to "Call when the water breaks."

I must say we were ready. The prenatal course was the educational advantage we had going for us. Prior to the course I had wondered about things like, "How's it going to get out?"

After the intensive training we received, I experienced other changes in my thinking. All of a sudden I began looking at gals as to how well they were shaped for being mothers. Also, there seemed to be a rash of pregnant women everywhere! On visits to supermarkets I found myself wandering down the baby-items aisle for the first time.

While we were prepared for the "worst," the actual experience was magnificent. Sharon started her final stages of labor about 7 A.M., exactly one week after the 3 centimeters' warning. I went to work and called at 10:30 to see how she was doing. "Five minutes apart," she calmly told me. After I arrived on the scene, we carefully timed the contractions. I had the impression that when it is for real, one could set your watch by the contractions. They weren't exact, though they were all under 4 minutes, so I wanted to wait. Sharon disagreed and called the doctor, who told her to come over immediately. I learned from this to always listen to the lady in labor, regardless of what the book says. The labor room was comfortable, and we settled in for the seige. Sharon's sister Kathy was the official photographer for the duration, including delivery.

Two and one-half hours later Kurt II made his grand entrance. Sharon, without any drugs whatsoever, had become a mother. It was a little while before I realized that this made me a father!

The memories of the original news, the nine-month wait, the classes, the "dreaded transition" that never happened (we thought at the time it was a harder contraction) form a wonderful background for the little guy who's come to live with us.

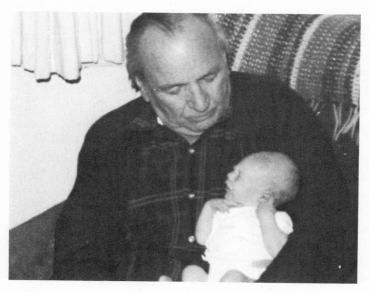

A grandfather.

"Claire, you have a little brother"

I'd like to start with the first experience we had with the birth of Claire, our little girl.

Neither one of us was very young when Claire was conceived. I was 31, and I was greatly interested and wanted to be involved with the pregnancy.

Ava went to some classes, and there was some encouragement for me to attend. I thought it would be fascinating to be present at the birth, even though I didn't know if I'd really go through with it. As it turned out, I was strapped in a wheelchair and told to stay out of the way when Claire was born. I was just there, and I kind of resented the fact that I was *there* at their convenience.

First of all, I would like to have been trusted not to lose my head. I didn't see any reason why in all that long time Ava was in labor I had to be banished from the room from time to time. Heavens, we'd been married for some time, and I knew what was going on.

When I knew we were going to have this pregnancy and I knew this time I could be part of everything, I looked forward to this birth, even though the first experience was limited.

I really had no specific fears other than the average worry in the back of my mind for my wife and worry if the baby was going to be normal. But I was prepared, had seen birth movies, had discussed labor and birth in class, and felt secure. You might say I was mentally prepared not to be turned off at the sight of blood.

I took Ava to the hospital at midnight on Sunday because she was having hard labor contractions 3 minutes apart. However, she was only dilated to 3 centimeters—the same as she had been for a week or more. The doctor suggested Ava stay overnight and have some Demerol to help her relax and sleep. Because Ava was sleeping, I went home and slept also. Then at 6:30 A.M. she called me and said labor had begun.

When I arrived at the hospital at 7:15 A.M., Ava was already going great guns. I was kind of disappointed because we didn't have to use the relaxation techniques or some of the exercises we had practiced. By 7:30 she was doing rapid superficial breathing and having heavy backache, so I had my hand on her back rubbing hard. I thought about it at the time, "I should be more tired." But I was so busy, I kept looking at my watch and timing contractions. It took about 2 days for my arm to unclinch after 2 hours of hard back rubbing. It certainly served a purpose, and that's what matters.

There was no point in time when I felt like the staff wasn't immediately available, so I was never afraid.

Before 8 o'clock Ava was almost fully dilated and felt like pushing. Ava had to push for nearly an hour before delivery and was really working hard. I got a damp washcloth and wiped her face and kept her on top of it. My first problem in the delivery room was when I realized that I had my mask on upside down. It amused me at the time that I was concerned about it in the midst of all the things going on. The nurses were very efficient, stood at her head, helped her breathe, and prepared the solutions and the table.

I was absorbed by the whole scene.

Ava said, "The head is coming. The head is coming." The doctor said, "Go ahead and push." As I looked over Ava's stomach, the first thing I saw was the head. I really didn't have much to do but observe at this point. I didn't resent the fact that I didn't have anything to do. It was engrossing just to be there and be involved with everything. Of course, there was the moment of suspense. When the body just came out and I wondered, "What's it going to be?" After I had a brief glimpse, as the head and shoulders came out, I knew he was OK. Son-of-a-gun, he was a boy! He didn't do much initially. He didn't start squalling or anything, just quieted down and didn't say much of anything. As soon as he popped out all the way, I looked at the clock to see what time it was. The doctor clipped the cord and handed him to the nurse who put him in the Kreiselman and wiped him off.

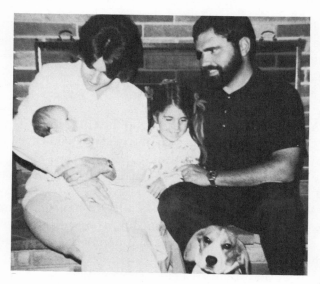

A family.

Then she turned around to me and said, "Here" I said, "Here?" She said, "You take him—I have other things to do." I turned around and offered him to Ava, but she was pushing out the placenta, so I held him. He felt very warm and seemed very satisfied. He was obviously breathing and comfortable and seemed very satisfied with the whole situation.

I was surprised they didn't have a scale in the delivery room. I was looking around for scales, and the nurses were estimating—I was anxious to know. One thing I watched carefully was when they tagged Ava and the baby. I wanted to be sure they were identified correctly. As I held him the whole time, I assured Ava that he had all his fingers and toes while the doctor was stitching the episiotomy.

After 15 minutes or so we went to the recovery room, and Ava held him then and nursed him. I wanted to tell our daughter first. She was staying with friends, so I dialed the phone and when the person on the other end of the phone answered, I couldn't remember her name. I was so high I said, "Who the hell is this?" I knew Julie's name, but for the life of me I couldn't remember it.

I told Julie we had a boy. Claire was standing right there and said, "Hello, Daddy!" I said, "Claire, you have a little brother." She said, "A BROTHER!" It was obviously a spontaneous reaction of real joy.

"A conversation between parents"

We feel a little high and shaky and tired. Our daughter, Sarah, was just born. She's a little giant weighing 9 pounds 14 ounces.

Stan: I'm so happy, and during labor you were wonderful.

Kathy: You don't know how it helped when I could look at you. Oh, I couldn't believe when I opened my eyes and a part of me was just hanging out.

Stan: Straight up in the air.

Kathy: Did you see her come out?

Stan: Yes, just a little white . . . he did the episiotomy. One labor pain you got her out about this far, then the next one you gave birth to the whole baby at once. It was beautiful.

Kathy: I think she's going to be a good baby, too. She has beautiful eyes and hands.

Stan: When you gave birth, it was after 13 hours 48 minutes of labor.

Kathy: If she came out that beautiful, who cares, really?

Stan: Well, she's a girl. We can definitely eliminate all the boys' names.

Kathy: Isn't that funny? I knew we would.

Stan: I kinda suspected. When the baby was born, I couldn't believe it. My eyes were actually . . . I was almost crying. It's so great. I went out to the waiting room to tell our families, but I couldn't leave that long, so I stepped out, looked around, and said "8- to 10-pound girl," and ran right back to the delivery room. That was neat with everybody there.

I just saw the most beautiful baby born today . . . probably in the whole world. Nine pounds, fourteen ounces. Whew!! When the baby was born . . . I never had that kind of feeling before.

IN MEMORIAM

When this manuscript was almost completed, it occurred to us that there were only happy endings in our book. We had been fortunate. Since statistically 10% to 15% of women fall into high-risk categories, accounting for over one half the fetal and neonatal deaths in the United States, it would seem that there would eventually have to be an unhappy ending among all the couples with whom we interacted. At last statistics caught up with us when a beautiful baby girl came into our lives for just a short time.

Following is an account of her short stay and what it meant to her parents.

"Jennifer Lynn"

They had her to love for such a little time . . . just 26 days. Her stay was so brief, but she left so many lovely memories.

The pregnancy seemed normal from the beginning, and in the last two months of the pregnancy Jackie and Al went to classes to prepare for their child's birth. They attended every class, eagerly read all assignments, and practiced breathing techniques faithfully. When labor began, they felt ready for it and went to the hospital together. The labor was long, lasting over 20 hours, progressing much more slowly than they had anticipated. Al did his best to support Jackie, rubbing her back, bringing ice chips and cold rags, and eventually found himself most useful as Jackie's focal point. As long as he was there to look at and to concentrate on, she seemed to be better able to use the breathing techniques she had practiced.

It wasn't until a few hours before delivery that there was any indication that something was wrong. The following dialogue belongs to Jackie and Al as they share with you.

Jackie: At about 2:30 in the afternoon I sensed an uneasiness. It was a weird, scary feeling—like something was wrong. I sensed that something was wrong with the baby, so I called the nurse and asked her to call the doctor and tell him. It was then that they put me back on the fetal monitor again and kept me on it this time.

Al: I was nervous, wondering if there would be problems. As I watched the monitor, it reassured me just knowing the baby's heartbeat was going. I could see it, so I at least knew the baby was still there, alive.

Jackie: The doctor and nurses stood by the door to my room, talking. This scared me even more because I wondered what they were talking about. They kept telling me everything was OK and not to worry. But the more they said this the more frightened I became because I still sensed that something was wrong with my baby.

Al: Some time after 3:30 I was gowned up and ready to go into the delivery room. In there I stood at Jackie's head to help keep her relaxed.

Jackie: I was still frightened, feeling that something was wrong. The best way to describe it is to say I felt like a woman must feel when she is waiting for her husband to come home from work when he's late. Then the phone rings, and she learns he's been hurt in an accident. She's stunned . . . the feeling is unreal. That's how I felt when we went into the delivery room.

Al: I saw her born. Her head was perfectly normal, round, and a nice flesh color. She looked so normal, but she never really cried . . . just whimpered. The doctor said right away, "It's a girl," and I said, "Whoopee!"

Jackie: When the doctor put Jenny on my stomach, all I had time to do was look at her, count her fingers and toes, and see that she was a girl. Then her feet and hands turned very blue, and they took her away from me and put her in an isolette with oxygen. That's when I became hysterical, crying, "My God, what's wrong with my baby?"

Al: Things went very fast, then. The nurses moved Jennifer to the nursery, called a pediatrician, and began treatment. This pediatrician called a specialist from the medical center in San Jose. I was trying to calm Jackie down and comfort her in the best way I knew.

Jackie: I don't remember much about what was happening during this time because they had given me a shot, although I do remember hollering over and over, "What's the matter with my baby?"

Al: By the time the doctor had repaired the episiotomy and Jackie was back in her bed in the recovery room, the heart specialist was in the hospital, having been flown over the mountain by helicopter. In the hall he explained to me that our daughter would have to be taken to the intensive care nursery at the medical center by helicopter and that she may not even survive the flight. After talking with him, I signed all the necessary papers and OK'd Jennifer's transfer. I'm so thankful that I was able to be there all the time because Jackie was still very upset.

Jackie: By now, Al and the specialist had talked to me in the recovery room. All I wanted was the truth. I wanted to know what was wrong, and I wanted honest answers. The doctor told me our daughter was critically ill with a complicated heart problem and a collapsed lung.

Al: All this time I tried to keep myself together in order to keep her together. I tried to comfort Jackie the best way I knew how in this family crisis.

Jackie: Because I insisted, the nurses and Al pushed me in my bed to the nursery so I could see my baby before she went away. You, see, I had a feeling she might not live, and I had to see her alive one more time. As they pushed her out of the nursery in a special incubator, I could see IVs hooked up to her head and her belly button. She looked so sick. "Take care of my baby," I cried, "My baby, my baby, I want my baby." I just wanted my daughter.

Al: It was strange. She wanted me to be two people—one to go with our baby in the helicopter and one to stay with her. I decided to stay and support Jackie because I knew the doctors and nurses could take care of Jennifer. In fact, I might be in their way. This whole experience has brought us a lot closer, all the way around. I won't say I wasn't scared because I was, but I wouldn't want it any different. It was such a thrill to see my daughter born.

Jackie: He was turning cartwheels at the birth because he had his girl.

Al: The next 2 days were like a dream, with our daughter miles away in an intensive care nursery. We kept in touch with her progress by phone until we could go to see her.

When they first went to the medical center to see their daughter, Al and Jackie found Jennifer in the intensive care nursery, being monitored and receiving oxygen by hood, intravenous feedings, and positive-pressure breathing help. Since they had been prepared for the scene they would see, they were not overwhelmed by the sight and sound of so much machinery. Again, they had numerous questions to ask, and they were answered. To be near Jennifer, Al and Jackie stayed overnight all weekend with relatives close to the medical center, and thus they could spend most of the first days in the hospital. Although they could see her and spend time with Jennifer right away, it was several days before they could hold her.

Al: You won't believe what happened when we first visited her. She was sleeping, hooked up to so many tubes and machines, and there was so much noise around, but I just stood by the isolette and said, "Hey, Sweetheart, this is your Daddy," and she responded out of a sound sleep. She squirmed and wiggled and practically turned cartwheels when she heard my voice.

Jackie: Al and I could feed her formula while the nurse held her, but it was a week before I could hold her. The only time I had held her had been those few minutes in the delivery room, so when the nurse finally said I could hold Jenny, I was scared to death. I cried and shook, and Al had to help me to the chair. I felt like I was holding a little china doll, like she might break. Al had to go out to have a smoke because he was shaking so badly. The nurse helped me and told me how to hold her and the oxygen, and then I did it myself.

Al: The first time I held her it was comical. It took the nurse and Jackie to get me organized, and Jackie had to be right there to hold the oxygen hose and wipe Jennifer's face. As soon as I got comfortable, it was all right. After a couple of times I got over the feeling that I would break her.

Jackie: By the following weekend I was beginning to take care of Jenny myself. Little by little the nurses showed me how to care for Jenny. They had told me that if I wanted my daughter home, I'd have to learn to care for her, and so I did . . . every day.

Finally, after 16 days, I was able to bring Jenny home. That was an exciting day. By the time I had done everything I had to do, we were just in time to pick Al up at work. Al came to the door, with his mouth open, white as a sheet when he saw us. I said, "How would Daddy like to carry his daughter to the car?" And he said, "Daddy would like to carry his daughter into the plant." So right into the plant we went with Jenny, as everyone gathered around. Al was standing there like a king, 100 feet tall. Jenny was his daughter. He was so proud.

The first days at home were difficult as Al and Jackie got used to Jenny's sounds and feedings. They were proud of her and showed her off to friends, even taking her to church on Sunday, smiling as people would say, "Oh, what a pretty baby." As the week passed, they became more confident in their care and began to relax with Jenny. She was a part of their family now. At the end of Jenny's first week at home, Jackie and Al prepared to give her a bath. She had been active and kicking and seemed no different than she had the day before.

Jackie: As I took her nightgown off, she seemed a bit limp, but I went ahead and gave her a bath, thinking it would perk her up as it often did. She kept looking at me like she wasn't feeling well. It wasn't her usual look, so I said, "Honey, call the doctor. Jenny is clammy." So we bundled her up, and I held her in the car on the way to the doctor's office. She focused only on me and seemed to be trying to tell me she wasn't well.

When they arrived at the doctor's office, the doctor immediately began treatment. Jenny's color was returning to normal and her temperature was rising when her heart stopped.

Jackie: Al and I were holding her when the doctor said, "Her lungs have stopped and her heart has stopped." I said, "Oh, my God, no!" She looked at me and at Al as if to say, "I know you're here, and I know you love me." Then she gave us a faint little smile, and that was it. I'm just thankful that we both were there because I never would have forgiven myself if she had been alone.

I refused to accept it and kept saying, "Oh, our baby, our baby," and held onto her for dear life. We held her for a long time. I knew she was dead because her body was cold, but I didn't want to let her go. She looked like a little china doll . . . like an angel, so beautiful and peaceful.

Jennifer Lynn was buried with beautiful services, emphasizing that she was loved from the time she was conceived, and that she always knew she was loved.

Jackie: After everyone left the chapel and we were alone, I picked Jenny up one more time. Al turned back the covers. She had such a pretty outfit on and looked so beautiful. We picked her up. She loved to be held in the left arm, close to the body, with the right hand rubbing her back, so that's the way I held her. Al put his arms around us, and we held her for a while.

Jackie and Al: When we picked that baby up, it was like the whole world was lifted from our hearts. She looked so peaceful and so much at rest that we let her go.

Jackie: Two weeks have passed, but I still feel like the biggest part of my life has been snatched away from me. I feel empty. When I see other mothers with healthy babies, I feel angry inside.

Al: It's been quiet around here. Something very important is gone. It hurts yet.

Jackie and Al: We knew she was on borrowed time from the beginning, but we had her and we loved her. We'll always have these memories of her. Some day we'll have another baby in Jennifer's room, to change that baby's diapers and to play with Jennifer's toys, except for some special things that will always be only hers.

UNIT V

Birth in retrospect

A collection of memories follow, as retold by fathers one to fifteen years after being present at the birth of their child or, in some cases, their children. Although most of these fathers attended childbirth classes, some of them did not.

In some families the fathers' experiences with the births of several of their children are extremely different, and these men are quick to remember and compare how they felt with each birth.

As these fathers reflected on the meaning of their participation in the birth experience, they expressed to us a great deal of satisfaction with themselves for having been involved and present at the birth, and most of them enjoyed reflecting and recounting their experiences.

"Each birth has been unique"

Greg is 15 years old now. We were living in Denver in 1961, attending the Unitarian church, which Dr. Robert Bradley also attended, and we knew something of him and his medical practice that included fathers at birth. We went to see Dr. Bradley after being turned off by a visit to a conventional obstetrician whose initial approach to us was to discuss pregnancy as though it were a disease or illness. At that time it seemed as though we were taking a chance on something unknown, maybe even leaving established medical practice and turning to something "far-out."

One of the first things I noticed when Virginia and I went to visit Dr. Bradley was that there were provisions for a father in the examining rooms. Obviously, he was interested in having me there, but nevertheless, I felt that I was invading a sacrosanct area. It was an area that I felt was private for women, and also it was an area that was under the control of doctors, and therefore I didn't feel really at ease standing by. I was part of the program because I wanted to be, but still I had to push myself to do it.

During Virginia's pregnancy I also came down with an ulcer, which complicated my attitude about being in the delivery room. Although I was looking forward to participating, I was not sure that I would be up to it. So I mentioned to Dr. Bradley that I might be a bit queasy in the delivery room. "What if I got sick?" His response was very positive, telling me I would be all right, and interestingly, I responded to his positive attitude.

Dr. Bradley had meetings for pregnant couples. Fifty or seventy people would show up. This was very helpful because I really had no idea about what was going to happen in labor and delivery. I still remember a film he showed at the last meeting. This film contrasted two reactions of fathers to a child who was having night fears. In one instance the father shook his hand at the boy, got on his high horse, and sent him back to bed. And in the other instance the father was understanding and not uptight or punishing. It's really strange to me because that film has remained in my mind ever since, and in situations like that I have a flashback to that film.

When Virginia went into labor and we went to the hospital, I still felt uneasy about going into the medical area—uncertain about what would be permitted or not permitted. But I had been prepared and knew what my role was to be, and so I did it. However, in spite of all our preparation, labor didn't go as we expected it would. Virginia and I began to get anxious because labor was slow and she was experiencing pain. At the point that I began to become worried, Dr. Bradley came in and spoke to us in a very reassuring manner, relaxing Virginia completely. The dramatic effect of that kind of support impressed me a great deal.

As we relaxed, labor moved more rapidly and we went into the delivery room. I was positioned at the head of the delivery table and had certain things to do, very much involved in supporting Virginia. The thing that impressed me very much again was the support of the obstetrician. I felt caught up into the spirit of it.

When the baby was born, it was absolute amazement for me. I saw Greg born from Virginia's angle, snapped my pictures, and remember being extremely delighted. The baby was put on Virginia's belly, but I don't remember touching him. What I remember most is that the really important thing to me was what was happening to Virginia. I saw my role more as support to her and her relationship to the baby. A lot of the care that was given to the baby was given by her with my support. My attitude at the time was that the care of the baby was the mother's role and my role was as a helper.

Although fifteen years is a long time ago, I remember some of the reactions I experienced from the people around me. If I would show the snapshots that I took at the birth, people would question if it was going to be a very good idea for my son to see these pictures later on. Would that cause him anxiety of some kind?

After the birth was over, I remember feeling very proud of what we had done—that we had pulled something off that was difficult to do. It felt very good. One of Dr. Bradley's messages was that going through birth together would strengthen the bond between parents instead of strengthening the bond between the mother and the obstetrician. And after this experience I believed him. I really felt that our birth experience strengthened the bond between Virginia and me.

Our second child, Melissa, was born almost thirteen years ago. During this pregnancy we were living in an area where no one was allowing fathers in delivery rooms. After our first experience we felt that we wanted to share birth again so we shopped around and finally found a doctor who owned his own little hospital and would allow us to do what we wanted. However, this situation was different; in contrast to the first hospital where Dr. Bradley had oriented the nursing staff to fathers' presence at birth, in this hospital the staff wasn't prepared for me. When it was time to go to the delivery room, the staff said I couldn't go in. It took a confrontation with the doctor and nurses to finally get me into the delivery room. Once inside, it turned out to be a difficult delivery and I was able to be a big help in coaching Virginia. Again I felt good about my participation but regretted that we had to literally confront the staff to have this experience.

John, our third child, is 7 years old and was born in this house. Home birth was yet another step we took after much discussion and thought. Actually, it was Virginia's suggestion because she felt it would be a more personal way. Even though we were able to be together the first two times, there were unpleasant experiences in dealing with hospital personnel—experiences we felt we didn't need. Although I did have worries about things not going right and our being far away from a hospital, I also was aware that the hospital was chancy in its own way.

This was something I didn't know the first time—that the hospital had its own pitfalls and chances. And so, being aware of this, it was easier to balance the whole thing—we were just trading one set of chances for another.

Each birth has been unique, but that first home birth was a tremendous experience. It was a stormy, rainy night, and one time the electricity went out. I thought we'd have to deliver the baby by candlelight because once into it, there was no turning back.

We had made arrangements for a woman to come and supervise the children, so that worked out well. When Dr. Miller arrived about 7 A.M., there was enough time for me to fix him breakfast, so we sat down and ate together. Then for the birth I acted as his assistant. This time I really felt that I was in my element, in my own home. It was my place, so I felt I was really a part of this—much more so than the other times when I felt I was sort of forcing my way into someone else's territory.

Immediately after the baby was born, the other children came into the room and took a peek at the baby so there was a warm, good feeling in the family. There was a rosy glow cast on this house, on the bedroom where the baby was born. The whole idea that this event had taken place here put an emotional charge on this place and the people who were involved. Even the woman who came here to tend the children felt like she

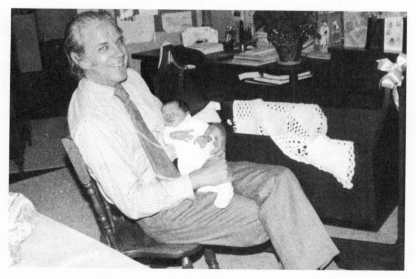

Enjoyed from the beginning.

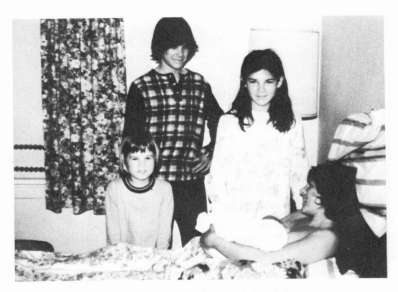

The Metz family on Nina's birthday.

belonged, although she had only occasionally been here before. There was an attachment there—almost like a grandmother.

When our last child was due to arrive two and one-half years ago, Dr. Miller had retired, so we contacted Dr. Whitt, who also delivers babies at home with the help of a midwife. Since we had one baby at home, I knew what to expect. However, this time Virginia went so fast that by the time I called the doctor, she was already in transition, so our son Greg and Nina and I helped the baby come into the world. This was a new experience for me and made me feel even more a part. I felt that the main thing for me was to assist in every way I could to help the baby come out and to breathe and then to wait calmly for the doctor to arrive. I certainly felt that I was an absolute necessity at that moment, and it has made me feel very close to this child.

I think my increased participation with each child has made me feel increasingly close to my children. An important part of my being with my wife at the births was to share an experience with her because I felt it would draw us together in our relationship as a couple.

Children are to be enjoyed from the beginning. They are people to relate to and to enjoy right from the time they come on the scene. It is fascinating to watch children explore the world, in the present, and as they grow up.

Also, I feel there is a protective angle in my role as father—to create a situation which is healthy from the time the children come into the world. Birth is a crucial time, and I could be active in helping them into life, not passive, leaving this responsibility to others.

It's a matter of deciding what's important, what's valuable. To me, family life is important, and anything which will strengthen family life is very important to me. My own experiences have been intensely personal and have made me increasingly aware of the possible influence of birth experiences on family life.

"Better than the best Christmas"

Five years ago our twin daughters were born, and I was there. How I came to be involved in the birth is rather interesting. When my wife went to see an obstetrician who had been recommended by a friend, she found that he encouraged fathers to come to classes on pregnancy and birth. So knowing this, I decided that as long as I was going to be a father, I'd like to be in on it all. My wife's encouragement really kept me going. Once we went to classes, I found myself really wanting to excel. As a matter of fact, some people in the class asked me if I studied medicine. I simply told them that I did my homework and felt like an "A" pupil.

The classes were large with 50 to 60 people in them and went on for months—almost through the whole pregnancy. After general lectures by the doctors we would break into smaller groups to practice exercises and breathing.

I still remember a funny thing that happened when labor began and we were ready to go to the hospital. We owned a small sports car at the time, and as we were leaving the house, Nobu said, "Oh, David, there's no way I can get in that car!" I had stashed away a $20 bill for an emergency, so I used it to pay for a taxi to the hospital.

When we arrived at the hospital, our training held me in good stead. Nobu was only in labor at the hospital for about 2 hours before we went to the delivery room. During those hours I rubbed her back and helped her the best I could. Then when it was time to go to the delivery room, I dressed in a scrub suit and went right in with her.

Our first girl weighed 4 pounds, 11½ ounces, and then the doctor made a comment that he was sorry this hadn't been diagnosed, but there was another baby in there. I was happy and grinning from ear to ear and so was Nobu. Then I told her, "I'm sorry, honey, but you've got to go through this again." And so she did. About 5 minutes after our first daughter was born, our second girl weighed in at 4 pounds, 4½ ounces. Because they were so little, they had to be put into an incubator. But first we held them for a few minutes; in fact, I held one baby while the nurses were cleaning up the other baby because there was no place for her.

It was weeks before I really knew I was a father. Well, maybe I knew I was a father—but not a parent.

I had heard horror stories about babies keeping you up for weeks on end, but our girls didn't really do that. Several nights one would be a little fussy, so I would take her and put her on my chest and she would quiet down. We didn't really have a hard time.

I do remember we had a log for breastfeeding. It was pages and pages on a yellow legal pad, keeping track of which breast had been used last feeding for which baby so that they would both have equal feedings. That was a lot of work.

Becoming parents changed our life-style totally. Suddenly there were two little beings totally dependent on us. I don't remember it being a frightening thing, but I know I thought about it a lot.

I never really got any reinforcement from anyone around me during the pregnancy or birth or right after it. In fact, I feel that Nobu and I are still pretty much on our own trying to do the right thing.

It's still my job to bathe the children. When they were infants and Nobu had so much to do, bathing the babies was one thing I could do to help her and be with the girls, too. It was such a nice time for us that I've continued to be actively involved in bathing them.

There is no doubt in my mind that the girls love me. I don't think they are afraid of me, and I see an awful lot of children whom I think are afraid of their fathers. Sometimes I think they would have reason to be, especially when I get angry and yell. But they aren't afraid. In fact, sometimes they even ignore me.

I've read books on child rearing and have tried various techniques, but I still feel that what kind of a father you are depends on what kind of a person you are. You can't be somebody you are not or use a method that doesn't fit you. Probably a large part of learning to be a father is just muddling through.

I've talked to lots of fathers who were very adamant about not being present at labor and birth, and they weren't. I don't know how I'd feel today about the girls if I hadn't been so involved. A lot of my wife's attitude and creative energy rubbed off on me and helped me continue to be involved. You see, she's a highly innovative person. The birth was something we shared, and although we still have our private moments about it, we do talk about it once in a while—still.

When I'm with the girls, or they sit on my lap, or they say something cute, or they're outside playing with other kids, I really feel there is just a little bit more between them and me because I was there when they were born. There are a lot of things said about babies not knowing anything in

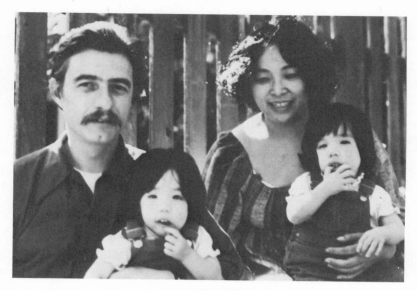

With the girls.

the womb or shortly after birth. Well, I don't subscribe to that theory. I think my daughters know Daddy was there, and if they think I was enthusiastic enough to be there when they were born, that has to make a difference in how they see me.

I know as far as my own feelings go, looking back on things, I can still get high on it five years later. There is a lasting, joyous memory—maybe even better than the best Christmas I ever had as a kid. I have forgotten a lot of them, but I've never forgotten my children being born. There are not too many times in a lifetime that you can have an experience so joyous that you can remember it all the rest of your life.

"One of the most salient experiences"

Our daughter was born ten years ago at Alta Bates Hospital in Berkeley. I was a student at the time, and we had heard about Lamaze childbirth through friends who had experienced it. Also Pat was concerned and fearful about what drugs might do to the baby. So we read books on prepared childbirth and were very interested in all the theories. Somewhere in my mind was also the idea that if Pat wasn't going to use any anesthesia for birth, I would have to help in any way I could.

During the pregnancy we went to classes on preparation for birth, held in a private home by a nurse who was also a physiotherapist.

When we actually got to the hospital, I was greeted with a little strangeness at the beginning. The doctor's later arrival seemed to serve as the catalyst to the staff's acceptance of us. After he arrived everything went smoother.

The classes we had taken had really prepared us well. I could rub my wife's back, encourage her to move around, and help her breathe. Now, ten years later, I remember having two emotions—one, I was very excited, and two, I wondered why it was taking so long.

Although I had helped to deliver lambs and calves, I found myself a little scared during part of the actual delivery. For some reason I hadn't expected to see so much blood. I remember being worried, not knowing if everything that was happening was normal. Then I would look at the doctor and see him apparently not concerned, so I was reassured by him.

When the delivery was all over and it was obvious that there were no problems, there was a great feeling of relief that the baby was all right and Pat was all right. I felt good about myself, very pleased to have been part of the process. It was something we had done together.

When our next baby was born seven years ago, the hospital rules and regulations would not permit me to be present in the delivery room. So this was an altogether different experience. It seemed to go on forever. I had to wait out in a room, uncertain and afraid as time seemed to move so slowly. When I knew Pat and the baby were OK, I again had a

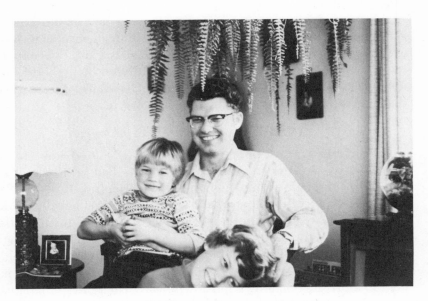

Feeling good as a parent.

tremendous feeling of relief . . . but it was different. I felt isolated, as though this experience was between Pat and the doctor, and I was kind of out of it. If I could repeat the second experience, I would choose a different hospital, where I could be present at the birth.

Looking back now, I realize that I had no preparation for fatherhood. Intellectually, I knew that I wanted children, but the reality of it— changing diapers and squalling babies was always in the future. So then when we had children, I knew very little about the whole process. In fact, it may have been halfway through the first Lamaze class before I realized I was going to be a father.

Being present at our daughter's birth was a high point in our relationship—my wife and I. It was one of the most salient experiences we have shared together.

I'd like to think we helped the children get a head start by not being drugged at birth. It makes me feel good about myself as a parent.

As I look back on those ten years, I find it hard to sort out my feelings. It was a matter of personal preference that we got involved in prepared childbirth to begin with. We simply wanted to avoid drugs and their potential ill effects on Pat and our children. We had no high-blown philosophical goals to begin with, but we ended up with a beautiful experience.

"No word can describe the feeling"

We never really did decide to have children. Five years ago we were told that because of an illness and low sperm count, the chance of having our own children was zero. We had checked into the adoption process and were scheduled for an interview when Betty became pregnant. We were interested in adopting because we both felt that children complete a family, and we could provide the love and care needed to raise a child who was without parents. We were extremely surprised and happy to learn we were to become natural parents.

We enrolled in a natural childbirth class consisting of six 3-hour sessions within a three week period. The class was held at a doctor's office and taught by a nurse. These classes were small in size and allowed for interaction between teacher and expectant parents. Through them we gained the knowledge and confidence needed to prepare us for child- birth. We are planning to enroll in these classes for our next birth. I read bits and pieces of *Nine Months of Reading* and *A Child is Born.* I was halfway through *Husband-Coached Childbirth* when the baby arrived.

When labor started at 2 A.M., feelings of excitement and anticipation to begin what we had been waiting for came over us. We started relaxing and timing the contractions, attempting to begin the routine of staying on top of the labor. At 7 A.M. we checked into the hospital and found the last 5 hours of labor had gotten us nowhere. The labor was then induced with Pitocin. At this point I was deflated to find the time before was wasted, but as the contractions became harder, my attention was turned to Betty and the problems at hand.

Around 9 A.M. Betty was taken into the x-ray room to determine if the baby was in an acceptable position to be delivered breech. Until this time we had been together, but I was not admitted into the x-ray room for obvious reasons. I knew my wife was understandably upset in this situation, and I felt very helpless waiting in the hall for her to finish. This feeling didn't last long because when I was admitted to the x-ray room, my wife had come apart at the seams. She was shaking and trembling so hard she was bouncing on the x-ray table and was vomiting.

When we returned to the labor room, she was given something to stop the vomiting and we proceeded to work very hard at getting on top of the labor again. This time was very intense, and the only feeling I can remember was concern to help Betty relax and gain control of the labor. In the next 6 hours my feelings ranged from ecstatic to below low and they covered hungry, tired, sad, happy, concerned, mad, and impatient. In retrospect, and after talking to Betty, through this interim period she thought we were doing terribly and I thought we were doing great. We were both probably partly correct.

At approximately 2:30 P.M. Betty was completely dilated and effaced, and we were instructed to start pushing. Looking back, I don't think any one person should be blamed, but after 1½ hours of pushing, a new nurse arrived and stated we had made *no progress* because we were pushing completely wrongly. Feeling? Deflated—both of us. Shortly after this my wife stated, "I'm going home. . . . We'll finish this tomorrow." Then she proceeded to try and get up and head for the door. I wasn't about to go through this again right away, so we pushed again, this time correctly and with good results for another hour.

No one word or words can describe the feeling completely—admiration for Betty, relief to see her face ecstatic instead of panic-ridden, awed by what I had just been a large part of, and over-whelmed at what was now bundled in my arms. At that point I didn't have a thought, but flashes of groups of thoughts, mostly . . . *we did it, life, healthy!*

When we were first at home alone with our baby, I felt proud, awed, and just a little apprehensive. We adjusted, I think, quite well because we were both completely dedicated to the new baby Jay. Aside from the loss of sleep, the change in routine and life-style, and Jay not having a bowel

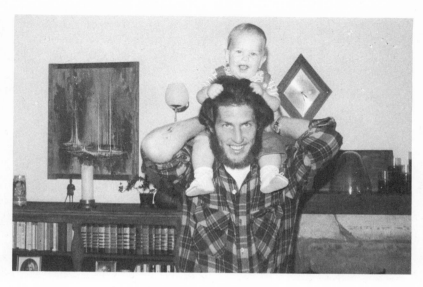

"I'm glad to be a father."

movement for 7 days and turning yellow, everything with him was fine. However, neither my wife nor I was ready for her convalescing period. Undoubtedly this is different for each mother and each birth, but Betty was down flat for one week and just barely "unflat" for the next.

The responsibility of being a father is awesome, but watching our son grow in the past year has made life even more worthwhile and enjoyable. I am definitely glad to be a father—so much so we are expecting our second small person in five months.

"Going home without the prize"

I had a friend whose four children all had been born at home, and he told it all so matter-of-factly. Even though I wouldn't want to take the risk of home birth, I felt that if he could be so involved in the births of his children, so could I.

So when Suzan was pregnant four years ago, I went to childbirth classes with her, feeling I could always back out if necessary. The class was an awareness in itself—being exposed to other couples who were expecting babies too. There seemed to be a cutting of the "taboo lines" by letting us know what to expect in the hospital, what we could do and why.

When Suzan was in labor and during the delivery, I got very involved helping her relax, encouraging her, and helping her push. Although at the

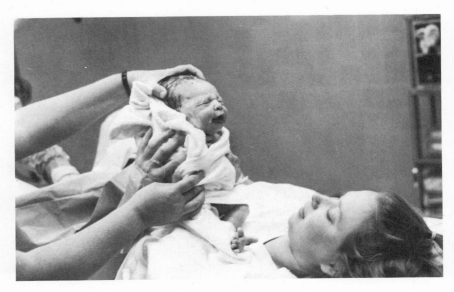

The baby was all right.

time I didn't realize how much my being there meant to her, later I learned that my support meant a great deal to Suzan. I suppose she had grown up thinking that the father would be out somewhere, smoking cigars and waiting. So when I was there with her, helping her, she appreciated me very much.

The doctor had set a mirror over the delivery table so I could see where the baby was coming out. But just as the baby's head crowned, he turned the mirror so I couldn't see. This frightened me for a moment because I thought maybe something was wrong. I still remember the fear I experienced until I knew the baby was all right.

Neither Suzan nor I held Tyler in the delivery room because the nurse put him right in the incubator. He changed from a pale color to pink very rapidly, and then the nurses took him to the nursery. I remember going back to the nursery to see Tyler, looking at him through a window. It's really hard to relate from 8 feet away. It was as though they were withdrawing him from me.

After I was sure Suzan and Tyler were OK, I went home, alone, and phoned everybody to tell them about the baby. That was the first night Suzan and I were apart, and I felt lonely and sad.

The next morning I went back to work, just to tell everybody. After a 3-hour coffee break the boss said, "Go on, go home." And so I went to see Suzan at the hospital, only to find her very upset and crying because the

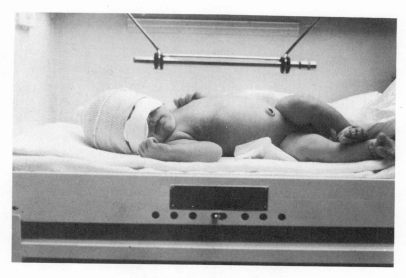

Under a special light.

baby was jaundiced and being kept in the nursery under a special light. It was 24 hours before Suzan could go into the nursery to breastfeed Tyler. We felt very frustrated, especially when we had to go home without him. It was like going home without the prize. When we finally brought the baby home a few days later, we didn't have the baby clothes with us. The staff was so surprised that we weren't prepared to take him home. Although it was almost an anticlimax after waiting just those few days, it was great to bring Tyler home.

Sometimes I wonder if I didn't start taking things for granted after the first baby. When Tyler was over a year old, Suzan was pregnant again. This time we went to a childbirth refresher class in a private home, and I wasn't as apprehensive or as nervous as I had been the first time.

Although we went to the same hospital for this second delivery, everything seemed different—the nurses and the room especially. Suzan had labored all night, so we had both been without sleep and were tired.

With this birth the doctor handed Colby to us, and we both had a chance to hold him. I thought then, "Why didn't we get an opportunity to hold Tyler the first time?" It seemed so different.

Again, with this birth we had to leave our baby at the hospital because he developed a respiratory problem. This time it wasn't so hard because we had Tyler to come home to and to hold.

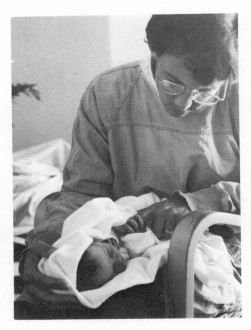

Dad and Tyler.

At first we were a couple bringing this new being to join us. This time we were a couple with a little being, bringing a new being to join us. We were a family.

"We were a team"

Janice came up with the idea that I might go to childbirth classes with her, and so I went, hoping I could be prepared for the birth and could help her. I remember that the class emphasized that Janice and I were going to be a team. The idea of teamwork was very important to me because I had played high school football and always been active in sports. Now we were going to work together to accomplish a final goal. I liked the idea that the husband would be looked on as the coach, also.

Once I realized that everyone in the class was doing the same thing, I didn't feel too silly doing some breathing exercises that really looked ridiculous. We practiced concentrating and relaxing and shared our practice with other people. But the total outcome we couldn't share because it was ours alone.

Toward the end of the class sessions Janice thought she was in labor, so we spent some time in the hospital in false labor. Actually, this made us more familiar with the place when we went back a month later for the real thing.

When labor was for real, Janice was calm and even though I was excited, I didn't act crazy like you see fathers do on TV. Labor was harder than we expected, and we asked for local anesthesia. That's OK, really, we don't feel that was any kind of failure. We were prepared 100%, but we only had to use 50%. This doesn't mean we lost 50%; actually we gained 50%.

We were a team, and I was there when my baby was born. I'll never forget! I have a special feeling now—all my own.

Becoming a father literally changed my life by changing my own personal goal away from myself to Janice and my baby. I had been a student, but now I had to make a choice on what was more important to me. Pursuing my student role and earning a good living for my family weren't compatible. It was just too much of a hassle. So I acted on my choice and stopped going to school for now. There will be many years ahead of me to still reach my own personal goals.

My family is most important to me, and rather than making my family fit into my plans, I made my plans fit into our family. You might say our birth experience changed my life.

Being a father is giving.

"I'm not a bad daddy"

We have three children, ages 12, 9, and 4, each born in different areas of the country at separate times in my medical career. When the first two children were born, I wasn't present at their births. It seems the circumstances each time were so different in many ways. The first time I was a daddy was not planned, and there was a certain amount of mixed emotions accompanying that birth. So when it came to the medical people taking my wife away into a back room to deliver the baby, maybe it was a relief that someone else had the responsibility. Perhaps I wasn't even prepared for having children the first two times. I know that I can say definitely that I really felt uninvolved with the first two, not just with their deliveries but with the whole thing.

But then during the time interval before our last child was born, a growth process took place for me that caused me to be more appreciative and want to know more and be more involved than before. Of course, there was also planning in this last pregnancy, which there hadn't been before.

During my wife's labor this last time, I was in and out of the labor room all the time. I remember how pleased I was with the gynecologist's understanding and closeness as a person. Although he and I are friends, we are not close friends, and yet he seemed personally involved in my circumstances, which I appreciated.

Even though there is a closeness between me and the people who staff the hospital where we chose to deliver, I found myself feeling self-conscious about everyone knowing we were there. It was uncomfortable having to respond to everyone's cliches and reactions at a time when I wanted to be closest to the most important person. Think about the number of staff members involved in a birth—the scrub nurse, the circulating nurse, the doctors, the supervisor, and the other personnel. It seems like there was always someone around, attempting to share in this great thing. For me, I could have done without so many people to relate to.

When we were actually in the delivery room, I tried to separate out my role as father from my professional role as doctor by mechanically separating myself. I made myself stand where fathers would be, at the head of the delivery table, keeping close to Sarah, helping her. I stayed put, acting exactly like I think most fathers would, with camera on one arm, ready to take pictures of the birth.

Standing there in my "nonprofessional shoes," I felt completely at ease. The doctor seemed confident, able to handle all possible complications, and so I didn't worry. For some dumb reason, in most circumstances, I have tried not to show emotion. Unfortunately, many times this works for me by my not showing happiness in a great outward way. And yet at the birth I tried to appear happy for Sarah's sake.

We really expected a boy and wanted a boy. Although I knew, scientifically, that one cannot wish the sex of a baby into being, Sarah was just convinced we would have a boy. So when the baby was born, I wanted to see a boy and thought that I did. Even when the doctor said, "You have a beautiful baby girl," I didn't believe it. For 30 seconds or a minute I thought he must be wrong. Then when the doctor put the baby on Sarah's tummy and I could see her well, I knew she was a girl . . . Anne Jeanette, I had named her.

It took a while, maybe a week, to accept her as a little girl. It felt a little foreign for a while, like maybe she should be a boy. During the pregnancy I had wanted to determine the baby's sex by an amniocentesis and buccal smear; however, when I had mentioned this to Sarah, she had reacted so strongly against it that I had forgotten about it. Now I found myself thinking that if we had another child, we could do these procedures to determine its sex and thus maybe control our destiny. Perhaps for a lot of fathers it wouldn't have mattered if the baby was a

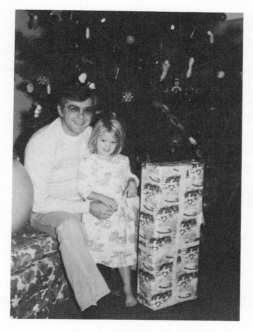

"Anne Jeanette I had named her."

boy or a girl. In my Lebanese background there is this big capitalization on having a male child. It's a big deal! There is a great family need to pass on the name by having more men in the family. It's vitally important!

Reflecting on Anne Jeanette's birth brings warm and pleasant thoughts that the memories of the first two totally uninvolved births do not bring. But I'll never be able to know what the experience might have been if this last baby had been a boy. In fantasy I've thought that to have a son would have brought total happiness, and yet at the same time I know that one single event cannot change one's whole life. I'm not a bad daddy, but I know I could be much better.

"Come on in"

Our first child was born in a military hospital in Germany nine years ago. There was no choice as to whether or not a father could be in the delivery room. I simply wasn't welcome, so I sat in an outer room with my mother-in-law and waited . . . hours. That was to me the worst ordeal of my life. Whatever happened in there, happened. Then later an orderly appeared at the door with this little wrinkled-up prune and said, "This is your daughter." It was hard to believe anything at the time. To see a wrinkled-up, purple thing wrapped up in a towel was unreal. Then the door closed, and this baby was gone. All that waiting and then an instant, "This is your daughter," and then taking her away left me feeling let down. There was no contact with my baby or my wife. The whole experience wasn't very fulfilling for me. Of course, I didn't care for that too much, but I didn't know that I had any other option.

The next day I went to visit my wife, and the baby was with her. I had to visit during visiting hours. It was a lovely thing, the two of them together. But then I had to go home again and wait until the next day to visit them. The whole experience never seemed real until I brought my wife and baby home to the apartment.

Then when my son was born four years ago, the birth was altogether different, even though I didn't get involved until the day of the actual delivery. I never went to classes or anything. You see, I never get excited about big, major events in life. I get very excited and nervous about little things—a door that won't open or a faucet that leaks. So I suppose four years ago that I just accepted the birth as a normal thing. I knew from friends that if I wanted to go into the delivery room, I could, but I didn't really think about it.

So when we went to the hospital to have our son, the labor went very fast. It seemed like only an hour after we arrived at the hospital Joan was ready to have the baby. The atmosphere there was so relaxed that I went in and sat down in the labor room. There were two young doctors, who said, "Everything is fine, this will be a lovely happening, come on in." It was just an invitation—like come on in and have a drink—very casual and warm. And so I figured, why not? It seemed to be the most natural thing. Why wait out in the hall and have the terrible experience I had before? So in I went, and before I knew it, my child was born. It was a most natural thing. I think that many primitive cultures have it way over our more civilized culture when it comes to birth.

It's interesting to remember now what happened when the whole baby popped out. I was waiting for a boy, and when out came the penis and he was a boy, I was jubilant. Then the first question was, "What's his name?" And that's when the name Kevin came out. Actually, it wasn't my choice—I was thinking of the name Jeremy or Joeffry. But I was so overjoyed with a boy coming out, I conceded to the name Joan had wanted. The name Kevin just came out, so maybe if I wasn't in there, the name wouldn't have been Kevin.

He may have been purple and looked like a prune, but I don't remember that. All I remember is that he looked like a boy . . . a beautiful boy. He stayed with us a while, was cleaned up, and we all talked a bit.

At this hospital I could come in any time and stay with my wife and baby. It was like walking into our own bedroom.

This time was a natural high experience that continued for the three days my wife and child were in the hospital. I even brought our daughter to the hospital to see her mother and baby brother. Then when I brought them home to our house, it was just a continuous thing. It seemed logical and made sense for us all to be there at home together.

I remember with the first baby, walking into the room and peeking at her, wondering if she was real. It was a fascination. But with the second child I didn't experience this. There was no surprise. The child was there, and I had witnessed the whole thing. It just seemed natural to bring the child home.

Being present at this child's birth was, for me, a natural experience. I was conscious of everything going on, sharing a very warm, spontaneous, natural event. There is an awareness about life that has seemed to evolve out of this. It has made me a much more relaxed person when thinking about birth as a part of life. Maybe up to that time I wasn't aware of what was happening. Just like everything else you never witness—you'll always wonder. I think that I'd like to be aware of my own death, not denied it.

Birth, death, life are all one. It's very easy to talk to kids about these things now. Maybe being present at my son's birth influenced that because how could I talk with kids about birth so naturally if I hadn't witnessed it?

"I had a family plan"

I had a family plan before I ever met my wife. My childhood idea was that I was going to wait until I was 25 years old to marry and have children. These plans were the result of my own childhood, in which the only children were just my brother and me. We were always happy together, just the two of us, and it seemed to me that in other families with lots of kids, none of the children got all the attention that was needed. You might say that in my head I always had the idea of what is actually the perfect life, and I think we've come close to it. I was very lucky to have found Linda, who has the same ideas I do. To me, marriage is a sacred thing, and that's why it was so important to wait and find the right person.

Our first child is 3½ years old, and we wanted her; she was planned. Linda wanted to have a natural birth in order to experience the birth. We went to only one childbirth class because we simply weren't comfortable with the group in the class.

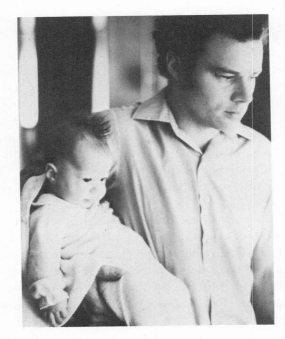

The perfect life.

Our doctor was leaving town, so he induced Linda with IVs. It was a long labor of 18 hours, with Linda in total control. During the labor I would give Linda some of my students' papers to correct and we talked. It seemed that it was best to keep Linda busy.

When the baby was to be born, Linda asked the doctor if I could go in the delivery room, and he said, "OK." I preferred being with her instead of sitting in some room, drinking coffee, wondering what was going on. It was comforting to watch this child being born. It was a really moving experience. In fact, I was so excited over the birth, holding my baby and all, that I even forgot about Linda for a minute. To hold my own baby right after birth was the biggest lift I could get . . . a natural high. The only concern I had with the birth was whether the baby had all her arms and toes and all. First thing the doctor said was, "She's a redhead, and she has all her parts." So then I relaxed.

I was so excited that I called everyone at 2 o'clock in the morning. When I went to school the next day, my students asked, "Mr. Baldwin, what's your baby's name?" And I didn't know. Well, they all laughed at me when I didn't even know the name of my own baby.

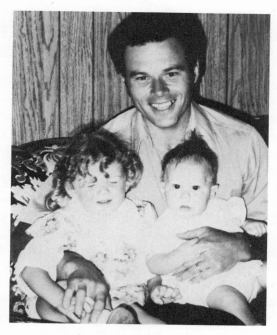

Mr. Baldwin's family.

Our second girl is 1½ years old now. With this pregnancy we went to no classes. Again, the labor and delivery went well.

When we brought the babies home, we kept them in the same room with us at first. Every time they sneezed, or coughed, or turned over, we woke up and looked at them, so we had few restful nights for a long time.

I ended up changing many diapers and have never been teased about it. It just seemed like that was the thing to do when it needed doing.

It's important for me to do things with my girls. After all, if you're going to be a father, you have to act like a father.

"Joy and jubilation"

When Jeff and Liz were born eleven and nine years ago, I really acted as an outsider. Also, no other fathers seemed to be involved with pregnancy and birth that many years ago. We really weren't expected to participate, so why would we even think of being in the delivery room?

Actually, I never saw Jeff for 1 to 1½ hours after he was born, and then it was through glass nursery walls in an incubator. It was the same way with our second child, except that lack of sleep due to a bout of false labor made us very tired at the second birth so that we just wanted it to be over.

By the time we were expecting Rebecca, five years ago, I wanted a different experience—one that would involve me and let me experience this birth. A couple in our church had their baby using Lamaze techniques with the husband present and told us what a terrific experience it was for them. So Karen and I talked it over and decided to attend Lamaze classes to prepare for a shared birth.

The total experience was tremendous. Preparation was the key thing for me, and without all the preliminaries and involvement ahead of time, I probably wouldn't have gone through the birth experience because to me, the preliminary preparation for birth was part of the birth experience. All the learning and sharing we did made me part of the experience—not just an observer.

This time when we went to the hospital, we were excited and ready to go as a team. What made the experience so fantastic was knowing quite a bit about what takes place during labor, and thus being able to help my wife and the doctor. I remember saying, "Push, push, now hold it," and seeing the baby's black hair appear, and then 10 minutes later, holding her, all wrapped up and warm.

Karen and I were crying because we were so happy. I remember counting all the baby's fingers and toes and asking, "Does she have them

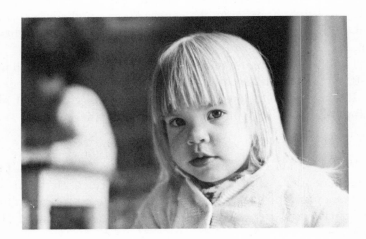

Rebecca.

all?" As soon as I knew she was all right, I relaxed. The aura of newness, awakening, and joy was so strong that I don't remember all the little details about the experience; however, I do remember the feeling of completeness that I experienced. I felt complete as a father. Because I was there at the birth and was active in preparing for it, there was a sense of fulfillment for me as a father and as a husband. The experience gave me great joy. The neat thing about Rebecca's birth was that I saw her so closely, from only a few feet away, for her birth and aftercare. Then when I came back to see her the next day, I recognized her, which was a different experience than I had with the first two babies. To get acquainted with them, I had to look them over closely on the day after they were born. With Rebecca I felt that I knew her.

We felt that this was our experience, not the world's experience, so we didn't take any pictures to show to others. Our experience was the feeling of joy to share. Maybe that's why some people have babies every two years—to renew a joyful feeling and to renew their commitment to each other.

Several years after Rebecca's birth we shared a similar feeling after we had worked very hard planting, tending, and then harvesting grapes. On our way home after unloading a gondola of grapes, we experienced a fantastic sunset, together, and felt elation and joy. After all the work we

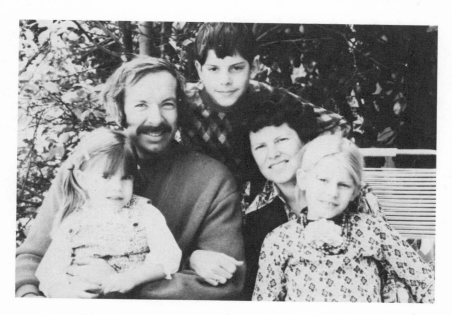

Everlasting joy.

had done together, it was like an applause, a final acknowledgment, a "well done." We compared our feeling to that unique experience we had when Rebecca was born. It was valuable, rewarding, everlasting joy.

Sharing in birth set me up to know that God exists. Experiencing this life-giving procedure was so profound that it was like walking on a mountain top, looking all around, and saying, "Man created this? No way! God created this. This is God's work." So it is when watching life begin. Life is the creation. The intense joy and jubilation that comes from the total experience of two people is so encompassing and so earthy that is helps me to understand my place in the world.

Epilogue

We have attempted to explore one group of men's experiences in pregnancy and birth. Although the birth experiences of only 33 fathers are included in this book, we were involved in collecting these impressions over a period of three years and have files bulging with experiences and photographs. It is tempting to make some profound statements and then follow with recommendations; however, since these interviews were not methodologically or statistically analyzed, we will simply briefly summarize. What we have witnessed has been heartening and offers serious reason for pause to those who insist on excluding the father from involvement in childbearing.

Over and over again fathers reported themselves to be profoundly affected by the birth of their infants and to experience a great feeling of satisfaction with themselves for sharing in the birth experience. These men's basic nurturing instincts seemed to allow them to find fathering both stimulating and gratifying. In fact, most of these fathers were just as involved as the mothers in interacting with their infants, although they often left the caretaking responsibilities to the baby's mother.

Expressing themselves in emotional tones did not seem at all difficult for these fathers—in fact, many of them wept with joy at the birth of their child. Although our work represents only a small sample of men, most of whom prepared themselves for birth, nevertheless it does offer insight into the feelings of fathers during labor and birth. Much work still needs to be done on whether new fathers of different socioeconomic-cultural groups have similar feelings to those shared with us. Knowledge of the needs of expectant fathers from other cultures will help us understand the father-child relationship as it influences all of us in the "family of man."

Glossary

amniocentesis Withdrawing fluid from the amniotic sac by transabdominal perforation of the uterus.

amniotic fluid The liquid in which the baby is floating in the bag of waters (amniotic sac) inside the uterus.

analgesia Loss of sensibility to pain.

anesthesia Complete or partial loss or absence of feeling or sensation, with or without loss of consciousness, as a result of injury, disease, hypnosis, or the administration of a drug or gas.

anesthesiologist A physician who administers anesthetics.

anoxia Oxygen deficiency.

antepartum Before delivery.

anterior lip A part of the cervix still gripping the baby's head. This corresponds to transition.

antiseptic An agent that will inhibit the growth or arrest the development of microorganisms without necessarily destroying them.

Apgar score A system of rating the infant's status at birth (the Apgar score is taken at 1 minute after birth and 4 minutes later):

	0	1	2
Heart rate	Absent	Slow, below 100	Over 100
Respiratory effort	Absent	Slow, irrregular	Good, crying
Muscle tone	Limp	Some flexion extremities	Active motion

Continued.

147

	0	**1**	**2**
Reflex irritability	No response	Grimace	Cough or sneeze
Color	Pale blue	Body pink, extremities blue	Completely pink

bilirubin The orange pigment of bile. This gives the yellow tint to the skin and conjunctiva in cases of jaundice.

breech delivery
    spontaneous breech delivery One in which the entire infant is expelled by natural forces without traction and without manipulation other than support of the infant.
    partial breech extraction One in which the infant is extruded as far as the umbilicus by natural forces, but the remainder of the body is extracted by the attendant.
    total breech extraction A breech delivery in which the entire body of the infant is extracted by the attendant.

buccal smear Microscopic examination of cells taken from mucous membrane of mouth.

cervix Lower, narrow end of the uterus.

cesarean section The delivery of the fetus through an incision in the abdominal and uterine walls.

contraception The prevention of conception or impregnation.

contraction A shortening of the uterine muscle.

crowning State in delivery when fetal head appears at the vulva.

Demerol Trade name for a synthetic morphine potency analgesic.

dermatologist A skin specialist.

Dextrostix A dipstick test paper to determine the presence of glucose in a liquid specimen (urine, blood).

diabetes A nutritional disease.

effacement The thinning out of the walls of the cervix until the cervix is drawn up into the main body of the uterus.

enema Injection of water, either plain or containing various drugs, etc., into the rectum and colon to empty the lower intestine.

epidural An obstetrical anesthetic offering a high degree of pain relief in labor.

episiotomy Surgical incision of the perineum to permit delivery of the baby without tears to the area.

fertility test A test that can determine and predict a man or woman's ability to produce offspring.

fetal heart tones The baby's heartbeat in utero. The normal limits of the fetal heart rate are between 160 and 120 a minute.

focal point A point to focus and concentrate on while experiencing labor contractions.

forceps An instrument used to deliver a baby.
fundus The top or upper, rounded portion of the uterus.

gestational age An infant's age determined according to the exact period of gestation. Weight serves as an assessment of growth and gestational age as an assessment of maturity.
gynecologist A physician who specializes in the diseases of women.

hematocrit The volume percentage of red corpuscles in uncoagulated whole blood.
hemoglobin The coloring substance of the red blood corpuscles; a chromoprotein of red color.
hypertension A condition in which a person has a higher blood pressure than normal for his or her age.
hyperventilation Chemical imbalance in the blood resulting from the flushing out of the carbon dioxide by overbreathing.

incubator An apparatus for maintaining premature infants in which the temperature may be regulated.
induced Helping to start labor with an intravenous solution and a synthetic hormone that causes the uterus to contract.
intensive care nursery A specially equipped newborn nursery where infants can receive intensive, often one-to-one, skilled nursing care on a round-the-clock basis.
intrapartum Occurring during labor.
I.V., intravenous An injection or infusion into a vein of an isotonic solution by means of a needle, catheter, and plastic tubing, connected to a bottle containing 250 to 500 ml of a solution.
Isolette A special infant incubator.

Kreiselman A mobile, explosion-proof infant resuscitator.

labor
   induction of labor The contrived initiation of uterine contractions prior to their spontaneous onset.
   stimulation of labor The induced augmentation of uterine contractions after their spontaneous or induced onset.

meconium Greenish black, odorless, tarry material in the intestine of the newborn. It is a mixture of mucus, bile, epithelial cells, and amniotic fluid.
monitor An electronic monitoring device designed to accurately record fetal heart rate and intrauterine pressure continuously during labor.
multipara A woman who has borne several children.

ovulating The growth and discharge of an unimpregnated ovum from the ovary.

paracervical block The transvaginal injection of an anesthetic solution on each side of the cervix.

pathogenic bacteria Organisms that are capable of producing disease in the body.

pediatrician A physician who specializes in the care of infants and children.

perinatology Special category of medicine caring for fetus from 28 weeks of gestation to infant 4 weeks of age, i.e., end of the neonatal period.

perineum The space between the vulva and the anus in a woman and between the scrotum and the anus in a man.

PKU An inborn error of metabolism of the essential amino acid phenylalanine. Without treatment, the condition usually results in mental retardation.

placenta The oval, flat spongy organ within the uterus that establishes communication between the mother and baby by means of an umbilical cord.

placenta previa A placenta implanted in the lower uterine segment so that it adjoins or covers the internal os of the cervix.

polyhydramnios An excess of amniotic fluid in the bag of waters during pregnancy.

posterior Toward the back. A posterior presentation is a baby lying with the crown of the head at the mother's back so that he is facing her front.

post partum After delivery or childbirth.

premature Preterm, immature infant, regardless of birth weight.

prenatal education Education for expectant parents before birth.

prep "Prepping." Having the pubic hair partially or totally shaved. Practices vary in different hospitals.

primipara A woman who has given birth to her first child.

psychoprophylaxis A method of training for childbirth, which stems from work done in the U.S.S.R. and France, based on Pavlovian theories of conditioned reflex behaviors and including "disassociation" techniques.

pudendal block An injection around the vagina, which anesthetizes the birth outlet. Usually done before a forceps delivery and before an episiotomy.

recovery A special nursing area where a woman is carefully monitored for at least 2 hours post partum—until her vital signs are normal.

resuscitated Brought back to full consciousness.

Rh factor A term applied to an inherited antigen in the human blood.

Rho-GAM Human anti-D globulin, commercially available since 1969. This material can bring about the clearance from the maternal circulation of Rh-positive fetal cells and thereby prevent sensitization.

ruptured membranes An opening in the bag of waters, allowing amniotic fluid to escape from the uterus.

saddle block The production of regional anesthesia, done only when delivery is imminent, by a subarachnoid injection of an anesthetic agent. This block anesthetizes the mother's perineum, the area that would come in contact with a saddle during horseback riding.

scrub suit A special suit worn by physicians and hospital personnel in areas where it is essential that they use all medical asepsis precautions.

silver nitrate Medication instilled in the infant's eyes as soon as possible after birth to prevent ophthalmia neonatorum.

"**special light**" A bilirubin reduction lamp used for phototherapy. Phototherapy changes indirect bilirubin into a water-soluble substance that can be eliminated by the kidney.

spinal block An injection into the spinal canal causing complete paralysis of the lower part of the body.

stirrups Special metal supports to hold a woman's legs while on the delivery table.

toxemia of pregnancy

acute toxemia of pregnancy An acute hypertensive disease peculiar to pregnant and puerperal women: called preeclampsia in its nonconvulsive stage and eclampsia in its convulsive stage.

preeclampsia Characterized by hypertension (BP 140/90 or more, a rise of 30 mm or more of the systolic blood pressure or a rise of 15 mm or more of the diastolic blood pressure), edema, and proteinuria, separate or together.

eclampsia Characterized by the same signs with superimposed convulsions and/or coma.

transition The end of the first stage of labor, when only a very small part of the cervix called the "lip" is around the infant's head.

tuberculosis An infectious disease marked by the formation of tubercles in any tissue, due to the presence of the tubercle bacillus.

ultrasound scan A noninvasive method that uses a B-mode scan to visualize the fetus in the uterus.

umbilical cord The cord connecting the placenta with the umbilicus of the fetus.

uterus A hollow pear-shaped muscular organ, the place of nourishment of the embryo and fetus; the womb.

vitamin K The antihemorrhagic vitamin complex that aids blood coagulation.

xylocaine An anesthetic agent used in regional anesthesia-analgesia.